[Not Just] A Little Prick

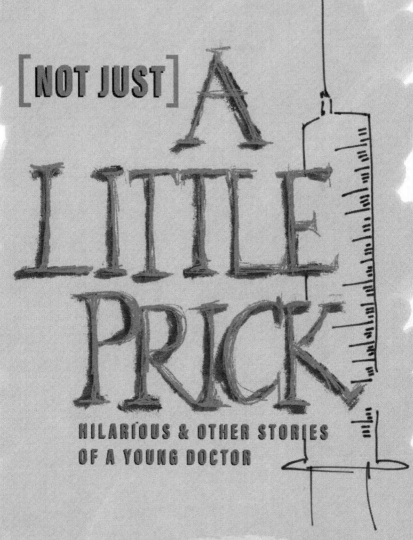

[NOT JUST] A LITTLE PRICK

HILARIOUS & OTHER STORIES OF A YOUNG DOCTOR

PETER DESMARAIS

Reach
PUBLISHERS

Published by Peter Desmarais using Reach Publishers' services,

illustrations done by Leonora Found
foundfive@icloud.com

Cover designed by Matthew Desmarais

Edited by Susan Hall for Reach Publishers
P O Box 1384, Wandsbeck, South Africa, 3631

Website: www.reachpublishers.co.za
E-mail: reach@reachpublish.co.za

www.notjustalittleprick.com

Contents

Acknowledgements

Thanks to everyone who encouraged me to write this book after listening to my stories over the years.

I am immensely grateful to my friends and family who read chapters in various stages. My aneasthetist and good friend PJ Allen not only read the manuscript, but had to endure frequent references to the chapters while we were operating in theatre.

A big hug and thanks to my immensely talented son, Matthew (who is a professional designer) for the cover that brought a smile to everyone.

I am indebted to my cousin Leonora Found who found (there I go again) the time in her busy schedule to do the illustrations.

A special thanks to David Gwynn for his encouragement and the time he spent with me proofreading the manuscript and making suggestions.

My publishers and the editors at Reach Publishers have made this a painless journey for which I thank them. I doubt if they would believe that the **entire book** was written with **one finger** on the iPhone. (Not the iPad or a PC, but the iPhone!) I had so many more funny stories, but my finger hurt too much to continue.

I cannot fail to thank Annie my lovely wife, my best friend and the love of my life for her patience and encouragement.

My deepest thanks go to the people I am no longer able to thank – my late mom and dad who made tremendous sacrifices to enable the poor boy from Newcastle to do medicine.

Preface

Every event described in this book actually happened and I hope that between Twitter, WhatsApp, Facebook and the rest of social media you'll find the time to read about my experiences.

While my stories are not all funny, I hope that when you next consult a doctor, you might recall some of them and remind yourself that despite the tragedy there is at least some humour in medicine.

A doctor might experience some of the most hilarious things imaginable and also frequently some of the most heart-breaking things imaginable.

Sometimes it's a combination of the above.

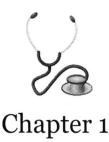

Chapter 1

What Is Doctor Talk?

What is "doctor talk"?

Medical doctors spend between six and nine years learning what some might consider an incomprehensible vocabulary.

I call it "doctor talk".

Like oceanographers and biochemists, doctors use thousands of unpronounceable terms and words composed of many glyphs with typographic ligatures that baffle most people and you get the impression that they are very smart. (I'm sure my reference to typographic ligatures rattled your brain.) When you combine the cryptic words with the poor handwriting, you should be rattled.

Still with me?

Well, does the following sound familiar?

You have a painful area at the back of your neck; so, you ask your spouse to take a look at it.

Your partner palpates your neck.

"Is it here?"

"No, somewhat further down."

"Is it here?"

"Yeah, but to the right."

"Here?"

"Yes, that's the spot."

"Gee, there seems to be something wrong with the joint between the vertebrae of your neck – perhaps you should consult a doctor."

So, you mosey off to your local general practitioner or GP and describe your symptoms.

"Take off your shirt and let's have a look," says the learned-looking doctor.

"Where does it hurt?"

"Just here, low down and on the right."

"Here?"

"No, a little lower."

"Is this tender?"

"Yes, that's the spot!"

The doctor frowns.

"You seem to have cervical spondyloarthropathy."

You're impressed – what a clever doctor!

Now, if you had a medical dictionary, you could determine that *cervical* is **neck**, *spondylo* refers to the **vertebra**, *arthro* refers to a **joint**, and *pathy* means **"something wrong with"**.

So, your doctor has told you exactly what your spouse told you: there's something wrong with the joint between your vertebrae.

This book is an account of my experiences after

expanding my vocabulary with the new words – I hope it won't test your ability to stay awake.

As a medical student, after seven years of training in medicine, you soon realise you won't be like *Doctor House*, the TV doctor, or the *Grey's Anatomy* actors, who regularly unbutton pretty blonde girls' blouses. You are stuck – the course is too long to go back.

As the Eagles sing about Hotel California, *"you can check out any time you like but you can never leave"*.

But it's a treasure chest of hilarity.

So why did I do medicine?

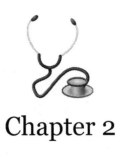

Chapter 2

And So It Begins: First Day in Practice

Fresh out of resident training in the summer of 1973, I took the plunge and joined Dr AG's general practice in Durban, South Africa.

It was a tumultuous year with the Vietnam war ending, and the Watergate scandal dominating our news.

Dr AG had the weekend off and left a memo for me to visit a patient recuperating from an aortofemoral bypass at St Augustine's Hospital intensive care unit (ICU).

An aortofemoral bypass is an operation where a surgeon uses a graft to bypass a clogged aorta (the large blood vessel in the abdomen that takes blood from the heart to the lower limbs).

The patient was being cared for by the surgeon.

My visit was a social one, which was just as well because I probably wouldn't have had a clue about the post-op care following this horrendous procedure.

Nine Augustinian sisters from France had established St Augustine's as a tuberculosis sanatorium in 1892, and it was now the largest private nursing home in Durban.

The Catholic origin of the hospital was obvious with a seven-foot marble statue of Jesus with his arms spread wide in the forecourt, but Clinic Holdings, a Jewish consortium, now owned and ran the hospital.

I gave no thought to this irony as I drove hurriedly past the statue.

In fact, for many years I had rather stupidly confused the identity of the statue.

I recall directing a patient to the hospital: "As you drive through the gates, you'll see a large statue of Moses."

The same patient saw me some months later: "I thought you said there's a statue of Moses? Boy – don't you know Jesus when you see him!"

When the Christians ran the hospital, the statue stood prominently in the centre of the forecourt, but the Jewish management later moved it quietly to one side.

With a large Muslim medical staff at the hospital now, the prickly question is whether they will now move the statue away from the hospital grounds altogether.

I turned into the gravelled forecourt, drove around the statue and parked in the doctors' parking.

Durban's summers are mostly hot and humid, and that year was no exception. It was midway through a sweltering Saturday morning and I wore an open-neck short-sleeved golf shirt and slouchy jeans. I passed through the double glass doors of the ICU and as the cool air-conditioned air hit my face, a stern-looking charge sister confronted me with a suspicious look.

"Where do you think you're going?" she demanded, stressing every word and wagging her outstretched finger under my nose.

Then she glanced down and noticed the stethoscope dangling from my right hand.

"Oh my gosh," she said, "Are you a doctor? I thought Durban High School had invaded the hospital!"

Although I barely think about it anymore, it was a reminder that my small stature and boyish looks might not augur well for my future as a doctor.

Those were the days when doctors did house calls. Instead of travelling to a doctor's appointment and getting other people sick, if you were sick you remained in bed and the doctor came to your house.

There were no calls yet for me and, this being my first day, I had no booked patients, so I took a leisurely drive downtown in my sporty yellow Alfa GT.

I had a classic black medical bag with drawers and compartments designed for doctors, a stethoscope and a two-way radio. When I was a hospital medical officer (SMO), I had a bleeper that drove me crazy. Now I had a proper walkie-talkie radio! (More appropriately, this is called a hand-held portable two-way radio transceiver with a "push-to-talk" button that turns the receiver off and the transmitter on.)

The radio crackled in my pocket: "006, 006, come in."

"006," I responded, pressing the button with the radio against my mouth.

"Are you anywhere near number 304 Florida Road? There's an old lady who has collapsed."

I was *nowhere* near Florida Road, but, eager for adventure, I responded: "Yes, I am – I'll go straight away."

I slapped the car into second gear. My right foot floored the accelerator and, with a vroom, the twin-overhead-cam Alfa lurched toward Florida Road – going right through a set of red lights.

Arriving at my destination, I brought the car to a screeching halt and, clutching my bag, I dashed through a rusty metal gate into a single-storey burnt-clay brick house. Weird sounds emanated from the back of the house and I hurried in that direction, from the passage to the dining room and through to the kitchen.

I entered the kitchen and confronted an elderly lifeless woman, lying sprawled out on her back on the stark linoleum, her brown eyes open and her lips blue.

She was obviously dead.

A young man was straddling her, vigorously doing external cardiac massage and a blonde woman (who I later learnt was the daughter of the lady) was giving mouth-to-mouth ventilation.

The ash-blue woman was unresponsive with widely dilated pupils, and you didn't need much imagination to grasp the futility of their efforts.

But the moment called for immediate action.

I placed my hand on the neck of the old lady and felt no pulse, but since it did not seem a good idea to dissuade them, I swapped places with the man. I coaxed him to do the mouth-to-mouth and snapped orders at the plainly distraught daughter to retrieve syringes and stuff from my medical bag.

It's at times like this that your hospital training kicks in.

Stopping momentarily, I rifled through my bag looking for a long needle used specifically for such cases. I yanked off the cap with my teeth and drew up an ampoule of 1:1000 adrenaline, which I plunged through a soft intercostal space overlying the heart.

As the blood gushed into the syringe, I knew I was most likely in one of the chambers.

Cardiopulmonary resuscitation (CPR) can be a painful exercise while struggling to find a vein, but I took a stab at injecting intravenous sodium bicarbonate into what seemed like a vessel in her forearm.

The reality of CPR is that it is physically punishing and psychologically draining. My neck and arms ached with each chest compression and I could feel ribs crackling with each downward thrust.

The rattle in her throat was off-putting, and I wondered how the man coped with his mouth locked over the old lady's mouth, her nostrils pinched.

Out of breath and exhausted, I reckoned it was time to quit, and I raised my hand for them to stop. The daughter stepped back and moments later the man took a deep breath, exhaled and stood quietly for a few seconds. I think he knew the chance of resuscitating the old lady was slim.

With a heavy heart, I steered the couple into the lounge, where they collapsed on an overstuffed couch alongside a row of upright chairs.

I left the sobbing couple and returned to the old lady in the kitchen, where I wiped the sweat from my brow.

It was jarring to see her lying there in her flamboyant floral dress with one arm at an awkward angle, her bare legs outstretched and a shoe lying a few feet away – ungainly like a rag doll.

She was motionless with white froth clouding her mouth, her eyes deeply sunk in their sockets, and I again noted the fixed and dilated pupils that had portended a grim outcome.

My impression was that she had probably suffered a stroke.

Witnessing death is a profound experience – something we try to stay as far away from as we can but the dead woman on the kitchen floor really got me thinking about it.

It bothered me that their dog, a light brown Labrador, had wandered aimlessly into the kitchen and stood wagging his tail and sniffing the lady.

I looked around for inspiration.

Then I realised I did not know what to do when someone died. (Not to mention the pathetic gap in my training where no one had ever told me how to manage grieving people.)

When a patient died in the training hospital, I certified the patient dead and the nursing staff took over. I never knew what they did.

They may have done what my mom always told me. "They put pennies on their eyes, you know," she once said.

As a doctor, how do you let on that you don't have the foggiest idea of what to do when someone dies? (The assumption would be that I failed to resuscitate because I lacked experience! Perhaps someone older could have saved her life.)

The dog, his tail wagging, was still sniffing the old lady, and I thought I should cover her.

I backed away from the dead woman and stepped back into the lounge where a slew of relatives had gathered, and I met each gaze in turn.

"I'm so... um... very, very sorry – but," I started, shaking my head, but I needn't have continued. My face said it all.

The daughter leapt up, clawing at her husband's shirt. Between sobbing, she gave a shrill scream: "Oh God no..."

She leant against him with her nails digging into his hand, a handkerchief in her other hand sopping wet with her tears. He said nothing and took her hand in his as she slumped back onto the couch.

I felt awkward, not knowing where to position my arms or what to say.

"Do you have a blanket? I need... please," I asked, my

thin, wavering voice barely rising above a whisper.

An elderly man seated against the wall stood up and promptly produced a tatty brown blanket. As he handed it to me, the three people sitting in a row alongside moved forward in unison as if to hand me the blanket.

Back in the kitchen, I stroked back the woman's grey hair and pulled the blanket over the body.

I felt helpless, but this little action gave me a feeling that I had just done something useful.

I squatted in the stricken silence wondering what to do.

Then I realised I had the two-way radio and could get help!

"006, 006," I called, lowering my voice so that the people in the lounge couldn't hear.

"Come in, 006."

"I'm at that house and the old lady is dead. What should I do?"

"If she's dead, there's nothing you can do," came the reply.

"No, no! You don't understand. I don't know what to do when someone dies," I said.

"Well, we are switchboard operators – neither do we!"

Then the voice added, "Hold on, we'll find out and get back to you."

After a few minutes, which felt like hours, the crackle of the radio scattered my thoughts, "006, 006... come in. We contacted Dr Vic Asherson, a Durban GP, who says you merely call the undertakers."

Well, how simple was that!

With renewed confidence, I stepped back into the living room, where more family members, some with their arms around one another's shoulders, had joined the grieving couple.

As I entered, the three people again moved forward inquiringly in their seats.

"Do you have a telephone directory?" I tried to sound professional, but my heart was hammering.

Once again the same three people leant forward in their seats as if to retrieve the book.

There was an element of humour seeing them move forward every time I needed something. It was like customers at a KFC outlet when orders get called out.

The son-in-law handed me a thick blue Durban telephone directory, and I flipped the pages to "Doves & Adlam Read".

I dialled the undertakers, who promised to dispatch an ambulance within the hour.

I looked around for a seat and wedged myself between two young women. We talked vaguely about their family and their kids, and I listened as one relative after the other, their eyes puffed and red, related memorable anecdotes of the dead lady.

It was a socially awkward moment, and I felt uneasy. Then for a reason, I cannot now quite articulate, I wanted to get away.

I bit my bottom lip. "I'm sorry, but I need to leave. I have patients waiting for me in my rooms."

(Cynics think that you're taught at medical school

how to tell lies with a straight face.)

The wife stood up and threw her arm around me. With tears in her eyes she gave me a hug and her wet cheek touched mine as I muttered, "I'm so sorry."

Then the son escorted me down the passage to the front door, his right hand just touching my arm.

"Thanks so much for coming," he said. "We don't even know you but you were great."

(Moments like this make medicine gratifying.)

He hesitated as he opened the door and cleared his throat: "Doctor, are you religious?"

Oh my gosh! My mind raced...

Did I overlook something? Should I join in prayer – or worse, lead a prayer?

"Well, I sometimes go to church, but I'm not that religious," I said.

"Well, doctor, thank you, because, while we were sitting there in the living room, *we heard you praying for our mom.*"

So, while I was speaking on my walkie-talkie radio, they thought I was praying!

There's a certain comfort in reliving the events of one's life. Some experiences are tragic and some humorous, but I'll resist the temptation to treat serious matters with levity.

Experiencing these events is like stepping into wet concrete – the footprint is there forever.

But you, dear reader, might want me to wind back the clock to see how I got to this point.

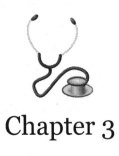

Chapter 3

Thinking about a Career (or Rambling on about One's Youth)

Newcastle in Northern KwaZulu-Natal, South Africa, nestles midway between the coastal city of Durban and the inland city of Johannesburg, which sprawls over the gold-bearing Witwatersrand Basin.

In the 1960s Newcastle was a calm village. Together with Amcor, the large iron ore smelting works, it had a curious mix of farming and heavy industry.

With its powerful industrial base, it was a place where one always felt that just a little more investment would have helped it to thrive.

Approaching Newcastle from the south, the road followed a gentle curve to the right then turned left to continue steeply down into the town, becoming Newcastle's main thoroughfare – Allen Street.

If you were a passenger in a car and looked down to change the radio station from Pat Boone's morose *April Love* to the upbeat *Jailhouse Rock* of Elvis Presley, you might have completely missed the town! (Or died trying – if you were the driver!)

This was unless you stopped at the only robot of the town at the intersection of Allen and Scott streets.

Had you, gentle reader, turned right into Scott Street and travelled a further two blocks, you would have happened upon an aquamarine-painted single-storey house with a silver corrugated roof and a simple front-porch right on the sidewalk.

(But if you carried on and reached the railway station, you would have gone too far. It was easy to go too far in Newcastle.)

This was 17 Scott Street, home to my parents, my older brother Paul, myself, and my little sister Margaret.

I think I had my first narrative memories there, from the late '50s through to the '70s. My two other siblings, Leon, 12 years older than me, and Cathy, 10 years older, had left home by the time we moved to Newcastle. Leon was a jockey and the South African champion in 1962. Cathy lived in Vryheid, Northern Natal, with her husband and two children.

The old house, riddled with termites and dry rot, had wooden tongue-and-groove panelled interior walls, which these days would be regarded as trendy.

It was reputedly the first hotel in Newcastle. I don't know when it was established, but it was probably in the early 1800s.

If you scraped away the layers of paint from the only gable blessing the veranda, you could discern the name of the hotel carved into the concrete. But I cannot, for the life of me, remember the name. Funny that.

The house seemed to be like a "woman of a certain age" – you know, in a state of perpetual indecision.

But my clearest memories of childhood spring from my life at 17 Scott Street.

I know many people detest hearing the details of someone's youth, but if you spare me your indulgence...

I read somewhere that there's only one letter's difference between a "yarn" and a "yawn", and it is often a long chapter filled with childhood memories.

While I realise it's all about me, you might need to know a bit about me to appreciate the chapters in this book.

It was Bette Midler, in the film *Beaches*, who said:

"Enough about me, let's talk about you. What do you think of me?"

(But you could skip the next few pages if listening to someone rambling on about their childhood isn't your thing.

Raise your hands – you know who you are!)

There was no comfortable way to confront the re-alisation that I was a nerd in the making. I think you'll agree, because of how I was fascinated by the story of David Livingston (told to me by a childhood teacher). His mythical status as a missionary, doctor and explorer enchanted me.

While not everyone deserves to know the real you, as you will come to see, more symptoms of nerditis soon followed.

At that stage, if you asked me what I wanted to be when I grew up, my response was: "I want to be a doctor, a missionary and an explorer. Just like David Livingston," which sounds pretty good, now that I think about it.

There isn't terribly much left in the geographical world to explore and I cursed on dropping my hymn-book, so the missionary trip wasn't likely to fly.

But the world was a different place during the early '60s when the cool guys were getting high listening to acid rock and dishevelled hippies made the news. Four young men calling themselves The Beatles appeared and I remember the popping and vinyl-scratching sound of *Love Me Do* on our radio and in the jukeboxes in tearooms.

It was also the time when women freed themselves, jettisoning their bras and girdles!

And, oh yes, dentures were commonplace – each of my parents had a glass of water on the drawer next to their bed where they kept their dentures at night.

Yuri Gagarin, a Russian cosmonaut, was the first human in space, but South Africa didn't have TV, so we couldn't watch this remarkable feat.

Computers, the internet, video games, and sexting and texting didn't exist, and it was painfully hard to keep oneself amused, particularly in the evenings, which could be excruciatingly boring.

Our neighbours had a washing machine with ringers, two rollers rotating on top of each other, through which one fed the clothes to squeeze out the water (and break shirt buttons). But my mom used a metal and wood washboard, something that can be seen on YouTube today as a percussion instrument!

The winters were bleak. Electricity was expensive so I cannot recall that we ever had a heater, but we had a cylindrical fire-based copper geyser, which gave us a sizzling hot bath with just one or two newspapers burnt in its chamber.

I once made a DIY heater using a "KLIM" baby food container that I split in half with the shiny inside acting as a reflector. I used a sheet of asbestos for insulation and connected a six-inch strip of electrical resistance wire.

If you hooked one end of the wire to the positive current and the other to the negative, a current would flow and the resistance would generate heat – and *Voila!* You had a heater!

I plugged my heater into the 240 V household socket. There was a loud bang with a blinding flash, and the house was plunged into total blackness.

My father's booming voice echoed in the dark: "Peterrrr!" This one word started low and crescendoed to roll the R...

The fuse on the pole outside in the street had blown, and it took several hours before a technician from the municipality could sort it out!

Newcastle had an overburdened sewer, and in some areas, I remember the tankers coming around at night to manage the buckets of night soil from the *kleinhuisie* (our toilet was outside).

So, as you can gather, the bucolic Newcastle was a rather backward town.

Helicopter parenting was not something practised in those days, and my parents, while supportive, never encouraged or discouraged my ambitions. They were poor and alas university was expensive.

We had a modest life and looking at my relatives, even as an eight-year-old, I knew how it sucked to be poor, but I never grew up with class anger or resentment.

My dad's pay cheque ran out before the week's end, but in my developing mind I never considered that having money could shape one's future, so wanting to be a doctor was definitely not a pecuniary thing.

In fact, although I suffered the lady of poverty, I thought as much about wealth as most people think about their knuckles.

My father was a miner, and already when I was in my teens, he had been medically boarded with pneumoconiosis and was not able to work underground. He was highly intelligent and, although uneducated, he was a huge inspiration to me. Born in St Pierre, on the Indian Ocean Island of Reunion, his mother tongue was French, but he spoke half a dozen languages and helped as an interpreter at the local magistrate's court.

While he was a strict disciplinarian, punishment was seldom necessary because living in that little town we had few temptations or alternatives. (We couldn't go too far!)

As I lay in bed at night, I would hear my dad coughing from the pneumoconiosis, but I don't recall him complaining.

Pneumoconiosis is a group of occupational lung diseases caused by the inhalation of dust from working underground and, since my dad worked in the gold mines, he got the form of the disease known as silicosis (coal miners got anthracosis). Because he followed jobs around, I attended nine or ten primary schools. But when we settled in Newcastle, he managed an open-cast stone quarry just north of the town and I went to the same school from Grade 7 to Grade 12 (Standard 10.)

I have a beautiful certificate that has nothing to do with medicine. It has a big red seal in one lower corner and is headed **MILWAUKEE SCHOOL OF WATCHMAKING – Diploma in horology**. It now hangs in my medical consulting room as a reminder of a childhood hobby, but also as a token of what eventually got me into a speciality, as will be evident much later in this book.

My dad used to tinker with watches, eventually becoming the town's acknowledged lay watchmaker and supplementing his income repairing watches. I learnt a lot from him and at the age of about 16 did a correspondence watchmaking course.

Lectures arrived by post every month and on two occasions a broken watch arrived by parcel post. I had to determine what the problem with the watch was and inform the school (by post).

Examinations were conducted at the local magistrate's

court and the diploma followed the successful outcome.

It's entirely possible that the diploma was offered by one of those fly-by-night colleges, because, search as I may, I cannot now find any reference to the Milwaukee School of Watchmaking!

But fixing watches helped to pay some of my way through medical school.

As a teenager, I had an uncanny interest in science and chemistry and had a laboratory in my bedroom with Winchester bottles of hydrochloric, sulphuric and nitric acid. (These were reagents that I obtained from a contact who was an acquaintance of a family friend and an industrial chemist at Amcor. Of course, hydrochloric acid – spirits of salts – could be bought from any hardware store.)

The bottles were each labelled with the formulae of the chemicals.

I was a puny kid and sport was less of my thing than academics, but even in those days it wasn't cool for a teenager to tinker in a laboratory.

But it was my favourite place to be.

The neighbours' children would catch frogs and my mother would give them a few pennies for each frog, then hand me the amphibians for experiments.

I made chloroform, which I gave to a frog in a bottle. Nowadays, you could Google "how to make chloroform" but I wonder where in the 1960s I found the recipe.

When the poor frog keeled over, I'd give it oxygen,

made by combining household bleach with hydrogen peroxide, to keep it alive.

(I'm sure, dear reader, you know this is the easiest way to make oxygen!)

I'd incise the abdomen and become transfixed as I peered at the frog's organs, but, while I was deeply curious, it didn't mean much to me since I never studied biology.

I used a needle with cotton to stitch up the abdomen and covered the wound with Nivea cream.

Some frogs died, but I moved the survivors to my "frog hospital" – a circle of wooden popsicle sticks stuck upright into the ground.

When a frog could hop over the sticks, I considered him "fit for discharge".

None of this seemed as silly then as it does now.

Isn't that weird?

I really can't say what my most transformational or Damascene moment was, but, as you can gather, it seems that doctoring was probably "in my blood".

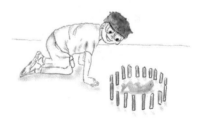

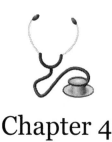

Chapter 4

Are Labels Good?

My petite mother showed little interest in my laboratory, so I was thrilled when, one day, she stood in the doorway and asked about the symbols on the labels.

She arched her eyebrows. "What does it all mean?" she asked.

It must have sounded like Greek to her, but I explained that NaCl was sodium chloride or table salt. NaOH was sodium hydroxide or caustic soda – a highly corrosive substance used as a drain cleaner – and $MgSO_4$ was magnesium sulphate or Epsom salts.

My soft-spoken mother crinkled her nose. "Why don't you just label the bottle caustic soda or Epsom salts?"

"No, Mom, we need to use symbols in chemistry," I said, with a hint of mischief.

"Oh," she said graciously, then lost interest and hustled off, muttering something incomprehensible.

Kids often know their parents so well, it doesn't take

much for them to read their minds, even when they say nothing, but I doubt if she understood.

A few weeks later, my father came home with a painful nail-fold abscess of his right thumb, a so-called *paronychia* or whitlow.

My mom, who trusted home remedies, told him to soak his thumb in a concentrated solution of Epsom salts in warm water.

She poured hot water into a plastic bowl and rummaged through the kitchen cupboards looking for Epsom salts, but, unable to find any, she said, "Well, I know Peter keeps it in his laboratory. I'll look there."

She trudged across to my bedroom and paused in the doorway staring at the bewildering array of bottles labelled with chemical symbols.

She ran her fingertips over the jars and pondered: $NaCl$, $NaHCO_3$, $MgSO_4$, $NaOH$... You can imagine what she was thinking: *Let's see, I wonder which one is Epsom salts.*

Her eye fell on a large coffee bottle with white crystals that looked like Epsom salts.

The label read "$NaOH$" (caustic soda – eish!).

She hesitated, retrieved the bottle and returned to the kitchen, where she scooped two large tablespoons of the highly caustic $NaOH$ (drain cleaner) into a dish of warm water and prompted my dad to stick his thumb into it.

His finger had barely touched the solution when he howled: "Shit! Betty. The bloody stuff's burning," and then in French; "*Merde* – I can't stand it!"

"Just keep your thumb in the dish. If it burns, it

means it's working," she said.

Unable to stand it, he yanked his thumb out. The skin around the nail was sloughing off and tears welled in his eyes.

"Dammit, what the hell is that stuff?"

"Well, Peter told me it was Epsom salts!" She was shaking her head slowly, distress etched into her face.

And then – *quelle horreur*! – to determine if it was Epsom salts, she opened the bottle and stuck the tip of her tongue in the crystals.

I got home from school just as both parents were returning from the emergency room of the local hospital!

I read that during the 1930s there was a notorious South African female criminal called Daisy de Melker, who murdered two husbands and a son and disposed of the bodies by immersing them in a bathtub with a strong solution of caustic soda. (While I suspect that the part of the story about dissolving the bodies is an urban legend, it highlights the extreme corrosiveness of caustic soda.)

Interestingly, Daisy de Melker trained as a student nurse in Durban, where most of the stories in this book take place. She was the second woman in South African history ever to be hanged.

And, oh yes, clear labels are good.

Chapter 5

Sibling Rivalry

Sometime later Paul worked up-country and arrived home one weekend with his eyes sore from driving into the intense sunlight.

"I'll get you some Eye-Gene," said my concerned mother.

Unable to find the popular eye drop in the medicine cupboard, and with me away at a friend's house, she said: "I think there's some in Peter's lab. I'll look there."

Without again considering how foolish it would be to take anything from my lab, she returned with a small dropper bottle labelled "Eye Gene".

(Unfortunately, the bottle actually contained methylated spirits, which I kept for experiments.)

Paul held his head back, splinting his eyes with his fingers, while she dropped meths into each eye.

"Shit!" he yelled and bolted upright, clawing at his eyes.

My poor mom kept muttering: "Oh my, I thought it

was Eye-Gene!"

I got home to find my grumpy brother had just returned from a visit to the local doctor!

(Let's be fair; it was another valuable lesson about labelling dangerous substances.)

I once made chlorine gas by adding hydrochloric acid to manganese dioxide, which is the black stuff you get when you split open a torch battery.

There was an immediate reaction, and I coughed and spluttered as the gas filled the room, choking the atmosphere.

I tried to flush the mixture into the drain but adding water caused more chlorine gas to form.

The yellow fumes spread through the house permeating every crack and crevice, and it wasn't long before the family had to flee and wait outside for the gas to clear.

It was many years later that I learnt that chlorine gas is a chemical agent used in warfare!

My older brother Paul, though fiercely protective of me, was suspicious of everything related to chemistry and it frustrated me that he showed no interest in my laboratory.

He installed a basin with piped water and a drain in my laboratory, but never joined in any of my exciting experiments.

On the last day of the high school term, he sneaked into the room.

I looked up to see him eating an apple as he stood quietly observing me making oxygen by heating potassium chlorate with manganese dioxide in a flask.

(If this description made you break into a sweat with flashbacks of school chemistry, I just wanted to see if you are still reading. But you, dear reader, might want to concentrate because I don't know why you don't know this.)

The gas bubbled through water into an inverted flask and Paul remarked through a mouthful of apple: "So, big deal – what's so great about that?"

Incensed, I quipped: "I'll show you the big deal!" and produced one of my dad's handbooks on explosives. (As Dad managed an open-cast quarry he worked with dynamite and other explosives.)

I flipped to the page itemising "Potassium Chlorate K_2CLO_3", and there, in bold letters, were the words **"Highly explosive"**.

He looked askance. "Well, why the hell are you heating it?" he asked.

I didn't explain the need for an open flame to combust, but smirked: "Well, *that's why* it's exciting."

"You're bloody crazy!" he said, aiming the apple core at my desk and storming out of the room.

A few hours later my mom opened the front door to two uniformed policemen, who had received a report about explosives in our house.

Paul for all his disengagement had sneaked to the police station and snitched on me. He reported that I was storing explosive materials at home!

He showed them the container with K_2CIO_4 and they cross-referenced it with the paragraph in the explosives book.

The police officers surveyed the laboratory and contemplated the chemicals.

What they saw bothered them, so they asked my mom for a container, and promptly put my entire laboratory into two cardboard boxes.

They drew a skull and crossbones on each box with the inscription "Danger" and carried the boxes to the local police station.

Much later, during my medical school holidays, I would go to the police charge office to see my laboratory – in two boxes on a shelf.

I wonder what eventually happened to it.

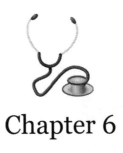

Chapter 6

Careers Week

In 1963, Newcastle High School and the Rotary organisation arranged a "careers week" at the Durban Tech, and I was a lucky attendee.

Durban, a large city on the South African east coast with a population of over 3 million (that's if you include the metro areas), is about 300 km from Newcastle and Africa's busiest port.

It has magnificent beaches, and it will intrigue most residents to know that it featured as one of the seven most magnificent cities in the world in a 2014 New7Wonders survey.

Bernard Weber initially created a project aimed at highlighting great natural and man-made wonders of the world and later included a city project. In 2014 the seven winners were Beirut, Doha, Durban, Havana, Kuala Lumpur, La Paz and Vigan, which kind of makes you wonder what the criteria were.

I have childhood memories of Durban, so I know

something about the place, but, having now lived most of my adult life there, I'm not so sure about the fuss.

However, the outstanding weather sets Durban apart. It has sizzling hot summers, with the colder winter's edge taken off by the warm Mozambique ocean current that cloaks the coast.

We were a small group of pupils from Durban at the careers week conference in 1963. Rotarians accommodated us in their homes, and I spent the week with a wealthy couple in Nicholson Road, Umbilo.

Those were prosperous years for Umbilo. The residents were affluent and magnificent double-storey homes were not uncommon.

My host parents owned a butchery and seemed to be rolling in it (*the husband drove a Rolls Royce, and his wife owned a fashion boutique*).

We were relaxing in the heavily draped lounge, where the lady offered me a bowl of fruit salad and ice cream.

"So how do you like Durban?" she asked, and suddenly a cockroach fell from the ceiling into my bowl.

What an embarrassment for my hosts!

The Durban Tech, at the top end of Smith Street, was an ornate brick building designed in an alluring colonial style, with an imposing bell tower and a classical facade that faced West Street. It had lots of steps and labyrinthine passages leading to the lecture rooms.

Built by the Duke of Connaught, the building celebrated its centenary in 2010 and seems unchanged to this day.

I looked at the conference programme and chose to attend a lecture on chemical engineering as a career option.

The students piled into the room, taking their seats while waiting for the lecturer and I spotted a scruffy-looking middle-aged man at the front of the class. He wore black-rimmed glasses and a dark brown suit that hung a bit large on his shoulders. He opened a shoddy little brown suitcase and pulled out a faded yellow Tupperware lunch box.

A murmur rose from a small crowd who were debating about telling the guy to leave before the lecturer arrived.

Moments later, the man glanced at his watch, tucked in his shirt, pushed at his spectacles with his middle finger and, clearing his throat, said: "Ladies and gentlemen, my name is Professor Black from the Department of Chemical Engineering at the University of Natal."

I made a mental note to exclude chemical engineering from my list of options.

I reminded myself that although we don't always have a choice about our circumstances, I knew with the conviction of adolescence that I still wanted to be a medical doctor.

But, dear reader, while you plan your dreams, the universe and especially the government might have other ideas, and nothing could have prepared me for what you will see happened at the end of 1964...

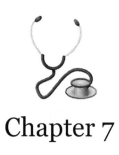

Chapter 7

Army

In November 1964 my life took a detour. I received my call-up papers; the government of the day's compulsory military conscription – national service – had caught up with me.

On 2nd January 1965, our crowded steam train headed for the dreaded Tempe camp just outside Bloemfontein. There were scores of us cramming the carriages. including two of my classmates, Rodney Collier and Glenton Barton. But with the coaches so jam-packed, I never saw either of them during what felt like an interminable trip.

It was late in the evening when the train ground to a halt at the rain-drenched Bloemfontein station.

A loudspeaker barked orders, and I scrambled onto the gloomy and wet platform cluttered with overturned dustbins and almost got lost in the melee.

We were herded into three mud-spattered armoured trucks, which sped off into the dark, leaving me with an overwhelming feeling of doom.

I wanted to run away, but I couldn't.

The Bedford truck with its canvas sides swung into a gravel driveway and through a wrought-iron gate with an armed guard on each side.

Looking back, I saw the gentle drizzle on their helmets and on the belted-wrapped khaki raincoats covering their shoulders, and I have an enduring memory of the falling rain and their images silhouetted against the moon.

A tear rolled down my cheek.

Would my suboptimal physical condition, and my five foot two inch small stature be an impediment? Did I fall short of the ideal fighting specimen they were hoping for?

Would they stop trying? These were questions I kept asking myself.

Infantry basic training is gruelling and brings the reality of war into sharp focus.

I'm surprised that I survived the initial three months, but I put on a brave face and did have some fun.

We looked forward to the evenings when we did not need to do dozens of exhausting push-ups and nobody told us what to do. One met the wrong kind of people, but one also made great friends.

And, oh, I got amazingly fit.

I could play the trumpet and it occurred to me that I could join the military band, so I applied to play the euphonium (actually I could barely play the trumpet and certainly not the euphonium).

But, as so often happens in the military, the application went astray.

After six weeks of hectic basic training, they mustered us into an infantry division of our choice, and I volunteered for three-inch mortars.

To be brutally honest, I wanted to impress my brother, who – whenever we had a scrap – would tell me: "Go to the army and become a man!"

But mortar training was by far the most physically demanding of all infantry. The baseplate weighed about 24 lbs, the tripod another 48 lbs and I think the barrel was about 46 lbs.

We took turns carrying the various sections, but I could barely lift any part, let alone hop onto the back of a truck with the weapon.

In wartime, soldiers would have to lug the heavy mortar and their rifle into battle!

Luckily there was no military combat at the time, but training was still rigorous.

In April they seconded our regiment to 5 South African Infantry Battalion in Ladysmith, Natal about 100 km south of Newcastle.

My experiences in infantry could fill a separate book but will detract so much from the ultimate aim of entertaining you with the stories of my life as a medical student and young doctor, that I'll skip most of them.

Since I don't normally swear, thankfully I won't need to restrain myself from writing the many profanities in the dialogue.

(Spoil alert...

My stint in the SA Army Band has relevance to my medical career, so I'm obliged to include it even with the vulgarities – read it with your eyes closed. Otherwise, turn the page.)

I was just getting used to the rigours of mortar training when something marvellous happened: I was summoned to the Commandant's office. My application to play in the military band had succeeded.

I would wrap up the last few months with the SA Army Band in Pretoria and I could not have been more pleased.

The train left Ladysmith at about 10pm and I messaged my parents that we would pass through Newcastle later that night.

Winter was banging on the door as the train steamed into a chilly Newcastle near midnight, stopping only for about 20 minutes to offload goods that looked to me like tractor parts.

As we pulled into the station, I couldn't believe my eyes: my parents and little sister were waiting. My mom was clutching a biscuit tin filled with her homemade *zoetkoekies*.

But the moment was bitter-sweet, with only a few minutes to chat.

As we pulled away, I glanced out the window to see my dad with his hand in the air, a wavering smile on his face.

The sun rose over the Highveld as the train stopped with a jolt at Pretoria station. I could not relax and had stayed awake for most of the trip.

Services School Military Camp in Voortrekkerhoogte, just outside Pretoria, housed the South African Army Band, and cramped in the back of a military truck, with my infantry gear and rifle, and boxes of army supplies, I made the 30-minute trip to the camp.

I had no idea that the bandsmen were proper musicians.

Most had studied music at school, and one guy even had a university degree majoring in music!

Yikes!

But it nagged at me: if they discovered that I could barely play the trumpet, let alone the euphonium, they might shunt me back to infantry.

And it screwed with my head that I'd had the temerity to say I played the euphonium.

I don't know what appealed to me about that instrument. Perhaps it was the name – after all a "euphemism" is just "a nice way of expressing something".

I took my rucksack and military gear to the bungalow and went to meet the euphonium tutor, Sergeant Spencer, outside the band hall.

It was chilly, and I stood there shivering with my arms wrapped around myself.

Spencer was a chubby blond-haired guy in his late 30s, with his khaki shirt hanging half out of his trousers and his hair out of place. I later learnt that he was sarcastic, a bully and reviled by the trainees.

An arsehole of note, he knew he could – and probably would – abuse his position and still enjoy protection from any riposte by the military rules.

He greeted me with an indignant snarl. "You're the euph. player?"

I took a short breath. "Actually, I can't play the euphonium," I said.

I felt sick telling him.

He raised his eyebrows.

"Are you fucking kidding me? How the hell did you get here?"

The portly Spencer had a weird habit of swaying and salivating when he spoke.

He leant forward with his right cheek against my left ear.

"Exactly what the fuck can you play?"

It was a heated moment, but what the hell – I decided that I would say I couldn't play any brass instrument and let him assume I was a fast learner!

The army is not a place where one nurtures scruples.

"I can't play any instrument," I whimpered.

"Oh shit! You're kidding me."

He lowered the boom. "Do you want me to kick your ass? How the hell did you get here?" he repeated.

Then the big gun came out: "You'll be shipped straight back to bloody infantry."

I dreaded the thought of returning to mortars, and the pungency of his language suggested that he meant what he said.

I eyed him sheepishly. "But can't I try?"

He stared at me like I'd just asked him to sniff my crotch.

His outrage mounted as he spat out his words, the veins popping in his neck.

"Try? Try? How can you *try*? This is a bloody orchestra, not a nursery. Shit no, you can't *try*!"

"But let me try," I winced in as brave a voice as I could muster.

My pleading eyes caught his gaze. He studied my face and sighed, then his attitude suddenly changed.

He shifted his weight, reached for the euphonium and handed it to me.

Now – if you have never played a brass instrument, you probably won't know that you need to purse your lips while blowing, or there will be no sound.

It was bigger than I imagined and holding the instrument roughly to my pursed lips (as you do with a trumpet), I made a sound.

"Try that again!" he said, the spittle dripping down the corner of his mouth.

I did it four or five times.

He sensed a positive trend. "Try it while pressing a valve," he said.

This gave a different note for the same lip pressure (embouchure).

His mood became less rancorous and, now impressed, he shouted, "Yeah good." But I knew he meant "Fucker."

He fumbled and plucked a scrap of paper out of his

pocket and scribbled the fingering for the C major scale:

0-13-12-1-0-12-2-0.

Then he pointed a stubby finger at the notes and goaded me to play the scale.

"Try this. If you can."

I could play it blindfolded but wanted him to think that it was new to me, so I played the scale slowly and purposefully – deliberately making an error or two.

Oblivious to the charade, the portly Sgt Spencer swayed ecstatically from side to side.

Then he wrote the fingering for *London Bridge is Burning Down*.

0-0-12-0-12-12-1, 12-12-0 etc.

He summoned a rakish grin. "Okay, see if you can do this!"

I paused to make the demonstration appear impressive. Then I gave each successive note fractionally more resonance – much to the glee of Sgt Spencer.

It was a triumphant moment and, waving his arms, he called out to the four players watching us: "Dammit, guys. Check this little fucker! The little prick has never played the instrument – but listen to him. Give the little shit a chance."

There was back slapping and high fives as they welcomed me to the band.

When I arrived at the camp with my battle-dress regalia, they nicknamed me "canon donkey." Spencer always referred to me as "little prick", but my close friends called me "junior", which, although it seemed to fit better, didn't sound as awesome as "canon donkey".

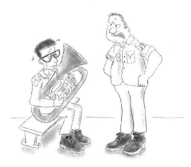

The Army enrols Army Band members with the Royal School of Music to study music theory, and I rapidly got through the first three grades (and Grade 5 at the end of the training).

By the third week, I was playing the euphonium for the State President!

Staff Sergeant Eric Parker (Staff Parker), a broad-chinned larger-than-life man, was in charge of the citizen force trainees.

He seldom spoke and limped like someone with a hip disorder, but I honestly never knew if he did have one.

He had Buerger's disease from years of smoking, so he may have had intermittent claudication.

"Intermittent claudication" is a rather fancy term for intermittent pain in the legs.

If you consult the medical dictionary I mentioned earlier in this book, you'll see that it's called "peripheral ischaemia" in "doctor language".

Here the demand for blood exceeds that supplied by the oxygen-carrying arteries – it's a matter of supply and demand. Since the supply may be fixed (by partial blockage of the arteries) and the demand may vary (say with exercise), pain may be intermittent. It's sometimes called Window Shopper's Disorder.

With online shopping, nobody window shops anymore, so I don't expect younger readers to know about this, but it was a favourite pastime in the 1950s and '60s.

A sufferer of lower limb ischaemia would stroll along the sidewalk and if he felt pain from the increased demand of the leg muscles, he could stop and glance at shop window displays waiting for the pain to abate. He could then continue walking until the pain recurred and again window shop.

I say "he" because it rarely occurred in women – probably because in those days, women seldom smoked.

I imagine that now with online shopping, we'll come across a new disorder called something like "Inertia-itis".

Staff Parker conducted the citizen force orchestra but played the bassoon in the permanent force band. He was subordinate to the director of music, Commandant Hewartson.

I notice that the rank, Commandant, has now reverted to the original British, Lieutenant-Colonel, in South Africa.

(I thought I might be starting to bore you, so I just threw in this bit of trivial information.)

When he learnt that my brother Leon was a champion jockey, he took an interest in my welfare and, as a happy consequence, I enjoyed many privileges such as frequent pass outs during my time there.

At the end of one's training, one has to perform a

solo for the Commandant, and I transposed some B flat trumpet sheet music for the E flat euphonium.

I chose a section from the Thendara overture and blasted confidently through the entire performance.

As I finished, Commandant Hewartson asked what I planned to do after military training.

I grinned. "Well, I want to study medicine," I said.

Hewartson put out his hand, "If you ever need a job, the PF band will have you."

So, as weird as it sounds, I had a career option other than medicine – I could have become a musician in the military band!

How embarrassing that at the passing out parade I got the Orpheus Award for the bandsman who showed the most progress!

I felt like a cheat.

Well, I really was – don't you think?

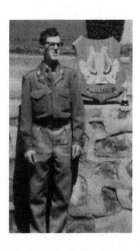

Here I am with the Orpheus Award I did not deserve. Ironically one of my pet peeves is people who fake their qualifications. I read somewhere that 70 per cent of Americans admit to imposter syndrome, but most people reach beyond their grasp and risk being found out for what they really are – frauds.

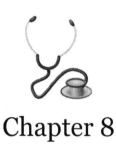

Chapter 8

Bursary

I'd completed my army stint. Phew!

But there was no money for medical studies. So I got a job – at a commercial bank.

Newbies start in the waste department, but, for some bizarre reason, they put me in the obscure and demanding bills department at Standard Bank in Newcastle.

I hadn't the foggiest understanding of what "bills" were and, despite having done accounting at school, I found it tedious and complicated, and I probably made a lousy job of it. I gathered it was another way of getting debtors to pay their debts. However, I recall feeling important presenting the bills to shop owners.

The job provided me with a rather unusual insight into the relationship of a bank with its clients, where vendors were polite to the bankers, often offering me tea and biscuits when I called to present their bills.

No one is proposing that companies should offer their bank refreshments, but the situation was a far cry from today's banking where – contrary to their fancy adverts – banks are about money, not relationships.

As my dad had developed pneumoconiosis from working underground, I was eligible to apply to the Chamber of Mines for a bursary.

I applied for so many bursaries that I hoped, relying purely on the law of averages, I would win at least one.

One afternoon, a letter with Chamber of Mines' markings arrived.

I tell you, man, my hands were shaking as I tore open the envelope.

"Dear Mr Tunguy-Desmarais," it read, "It is my pleasure to inform you that you are on the final selection list for one of six bursaries offered by the Chamber of Mines for students to study at a South African University."

Reading this, I had a smile that could light up a room and my heart leapt!

My parents took me to the bursary selection in Johannesburg, and we did the six-hour trip from Newcastle in my dad's blue 1961 Renault Dauphine.

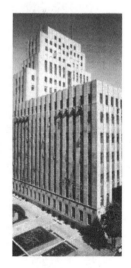

It was an arduous drive through the congested city to the Chamber of Mines' striking Art Deco building just off Holland Street, where the interview was held.

So, there I was, sitting with eleven other kids waiting in the foyer on the second floor of the building for the shootout: six places and a dozen kids... A 50/50 situation!

We sat perched on upright metal chairs in a circle with our legs crossed, waiting for the call.

A clock on the wall ticked.

The fan beat the air, and someone tapped a shoe restlessly against his chair.

My mind wandered as I assessed the nervous-looking candidates.

Clearing my throat, I asked a tall dark-haired guy opposite me: "What you gonna study?"

"Mining engineering," he mumbled.

I turned to the short freckle-faced boy next to me, who had not moved a muscle since we'd sat down, and asked, "And you?"

He glanced at me, smiled and then with a smug expression said: "Mining engineering, of course." I envied his optimism.

I pointed my index finger at the boy with a school blazer and black-rimmed spectacles. He was chatting to the guy next to him, but paused and said, "Geological engineering," then carried on with his conversation.

So, one was doing mining engineering, another mining engineering, another geology. Sounded like a version of the old one potato, two potato game.

Shit! I shuddered at the thought that the likelihood of a mining company giving a bursary to study medicine was slim!

I needed it or I would be stuck in that tiny bank forever.

They called my name and, with my eyes lowered, I crossed the tiled floor, passing through an ornate wooden door frame into a large conference room.

The interviewers were six men and a tall thin blonde-haired woman, all sitting around a shiny half-round table. I sat along the straight edge opposite them.

Behind them and lining one wall were bookcases housing gilt-edged leather-bound volumes and I breathed in the faint smells of glue in the spines of the books.

The room was suffused with a soft golden light, but the heavy gilt-framed artwork gave it a menacing feeling.

Just being there terrified me, but a younger fresh-faced man (who I later established was a top executive at the chamber) put me at ease with a smile and a greeting.

"I see you are from Newcastle," he said. "It's a long way away. We won't take up much of your time. Please relax."

An older man with rugged features and a greying moustache cleared his throat, "Desmarais... that's an unusual surname... could you be related to a Frenchman, Desmarais, who worked on Crown Mines in the 1930s?"

"Well, that could be my dad who worked underground on those mines," I answered.

There was a roar of laughter as the older man related an amusing story of "the crazy Frenchman", who swore at the African labourers in French.

The atmosphere was instantly more relaxed, and then, pointing to his right, he said: "Do you know Prof. Arthur Bleksley?"

Anybody in South Africa who had ever tuned in to the radio would have known Prof. Bleksley, professor of mathematics at the University of the Witwatersrand.

He was one of the *Three Wise Men* on the Thursday evening Springbok Radio quiz show, *Test The Team*. Listeners would send in tough questions hoping to stump the learned panel.

Apart from being a mathematics professor, Bleksley was also a world-renowned astronomer. He had a quick mind and a great sense of humour.

The three wise men were the Google of the 1960s and seemingly knew everything there was to know.

"Yes," I said, but I had never laid eyes on Bleksley. I had only heard him on Springbok Radio.

But Prof. Bleksley was sitting an arm's length in front of me and the voice was familiar.

As I was a card-carrying nerd, this radio personality dazzled me.

"Mr Desmarais," he said, "I see from your resume you play a musical instrument called a euphonium. What is this?"

I was amazed that Arthur Bleksley (the wise man of radio) did not know what a euphonium was!

"Well, it's a brass instrument – a kind of tuba. You'd more likely find it in a military band."

"A tuba! How can a little guy like you play an instrument as big as a tuba?"

"Well, I played it in the Army Band, where you march with it," I replied.

He tilted back in his chair and the veins on his neck popped out as he laughed.

Feeling more at ease, I relaxed my posture.

"Tell me, Mr Desmarais, if you won this bursary to study medicine, where would you enrol for the degree?"

"Well, the first year – basic sciences – at the University of Natal, either Durban or Pietermaritzburg. The subsequent years at Wits," I answered.

His eyes narrowed slightly, focusing on me intently.

"No, no. You must do all the years at one university," he said.

I was not sure how I'd missed that point and sat a little straighter. "Well then, I'll apply to Wits." (The name "Wits" is short for the University of the Witwatersrand – an English-medium university in Johannesburg.)

Then the tall blonde woman stood up, smacked her lips and said: "Wits selects students for the first year of study towards the degree of MB BCh during November of the year before. They base the selection on the candidates' matriculation results – I'm afraid the applications are already closed."

(I later learnt that she represented the University of the Witwatersrand.)

This was it for me – I moved my hand from my lap to my neck, pulled on my collar, shut my eyes and took a breath.

There was a deadly pause, then Prof. Bleksley spoke up.

"Why don't you apply to the University of Pretoria? They select the best students for medicine only after the first year, so you can apply for admission to the first year."

I turned to face him, picked at my fingernails and shrugged. "But it's an Afrikaans university," I stammered.

I hadn't mentioned that my mother's family was Afrikaans, so I could speak it well and had considered studying veterinary science at Pretoria as my second choice.

He tilted back in his seat, "Well, can't you speak Afrikaans?"

"Yeah, I can," I admitted.

The lady stood up again, with a small writing pad in her hand and announced, in exhaustive detail, that Pretoria University was registering their first-year students that day and the next, so there was not much time.

Bleksley made some ticks on a folio, then, after a strained moment, turned and, pounding his fist on the table, growled: "*Ry, Boeta, ry!*"

(This is Afrikaans for "Ride, my boy, ride!")

They ushered me out, and I left the building through a side door.

My mom and dad were sitting in the Renault parked under a tree, in the gardens of the Chamber buildings. The front passenger door was open, and my mom had taken out a thermos flask with tea.

As I approached, my dad called out, "Did you get the bursary?"

Although I didn't have a definite answer, I thought "*Ry, Boeta, ry*" might mean that I indeed had.

"You're going to get your dream!" my elated dad said, and we drove straight to Pretoria to register for MB ChB 1 at TUKs.

(TUKs, another name for the University of Pretoria, is an acronym derived from its original name, Transvaal University College, which was established in 1908.)

A week later, a thin brown envelope with the markings of the SA Chamber of Mines arrived, and I opened it with quivering hands and read: "It is with great pleasure that I inform you that the Chamber of Mines has awarded you a bursary for six years to read for the degree of MB ChB at the University of Pretoria."

This was the moment I knew for sure that I would be a doctor. I was excited and happy.

I needed to tell the bank about my plans, and the allure of a medical career.

I *was swapping a pay-cheque-at-the-end-of-the-day job for a vocation with purpose in my life.*

The bank had already shut its doors when I got to the manager and, with my heart pounding, I told him about my university decision.

"That's great, I love it when staff further their studies," he said. "Will you study by correspondence with the University of South Africa? BCom in Banking?"

"No, sir – I want to go to medical school to become a doctor," I said.

He laughed himself into a coughing fit and almost fell off his chair.

"A doctor! Are you out of your mind? Bankers don't become doctors. They study commerce and finance!"

While I know it's a cliché that good financial knowledge can be a great boom, I only realise it now – after 50 years.

The bursary was like winning the lottery. It covered tuition fees, books, instruments, accommodation and R150 pocket money every three months (a sizable amount of money in the '60s).

I was getting a full ride.

There was a condition: I could not fail *any* subject of *any* year.

It was Colin Powell who years later said:

"A dream doesn't become a reality through magic; it takes sweat, determination, and hard work."

But you have to give your dream a chance to come true.

I harboured no illusions as to the pressure I would be under to achieve this dream, but was I prepared for it?

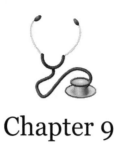

Chapter 9

Pretoria University-College Te Huis

T he Vietnam war was raging when I started my first year at the University of Pretoria in 1966, but I paid little attention to this.

I realise now that when you absorb yourself in your studies, you stubbornly shut your mind to events happening around you. The daily events making the news were the furthest things from my mind.

In the first year, the subjects chemistry, physics, botany and zoology were taken on the main campus, with the later pre-clinical training held at the building for Basic Medical Sciences (BMW Gebou – *Basiese Mediese Wetenskape*) at the top of Beatrix Street, quite a distance from the main campus.

Doing medicine at the University of Pretoria allowed first-year students liberal admission criteria and, at the end of the year, they ushered the 180 best students into the second year of medicine, where the clinical years followed at the Academic Hospital.

Pretoria is the administrative capital of South Africa, also called "Jacaranda city" because of the many jacaranda tree-lined streets.

In spring, the thousands of purple petals bespeckled the concrete and tar and we could hear the crackle and hiss as the cars' tyres crushed the flowers. If by luck a Jacaranda flower dropped on your head on the day of an exam, it was a sure sign you would pass the exam!

(There is presently a rigorous debate about protecting the Jacaranda trees, which are not indigenous to the area.)

I savoured the time I spent studying in the gardens of the imposing Union Buildings, which are situated at the highest point of the city and which define Pretoria.

Sir Herbert Baker, the architect of South Africa House in London's Trafalgar Square, designed the buildings to celebrate the merger of the four provinces to form the Union of South Africa in 1910.

Not much exciting ever happened in Pretoria, but, with its temperate climate, it was an ideal city in which to study. But I guess it's also likely that the lack of distractions was a better reason (especially if you were a nerd).

If one chose to let one's hair down and be silly, one could take the 40-minute drive to the hustle and bustle of Johannesburg with its exciting nightlife.

Why it took so long is a mystery because these days

it's a 20-minute trip by car and it is inconceivable that Pretoria has magically moved closer to Johannesburg since the 1960s.

But Joeys was where there was never-ending excitement.

I found accommodation at College Te Huis students' residence, a residence notorious for the harsh initiation (*ontgroening*) of first-year students.

I don't want to be scathing about my time at College Te Huis and I wish I could say it was fun – but I would be lying.

As part of the initiation, the senior students insisted that as first-year students we carry large cardboard signs dangling from our necks, with the details of the degree and courses for which we had enrolled listed.

If we had indicated medicine or veterinary science, then we had to show what we intended to study the following year (the assumption being that we would most likely not get selected for the second year of the course we were registered for).

In addition, we listed our supposedly good and bad attributes.

We had to display this demeaning sign whenever we left our room and at all mealtimes. We even had to wear it while in the toilet or bath.

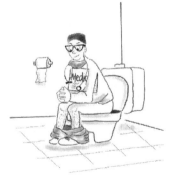

A senior would wake us at 5am, and line us up in front of the residence to perform childish acts for the amusement of the people hurrying along the sidewalk.

We endured impassive and rude stares from passing workmen in their greasy overalls while we dictated and acted out a poem that the seniors had composed. It was in Afrikaans, but here it is translated (most of this will not make sense written).

"*On my father's farm, there are many dogs. There are small dogs* [then we raised our arms above our heads, i.e. the opposite] *and large dogs* [then gesturing small]. *There are thin dogs* [spread our arms wide] *and fat dogs* [holding our hands only slightly apart], *but the best dog of all is Woofie the collie dog.*"

I winced when we had to go down on all fours and yap at each other's backsides, reciting: "*Woofie die kollie hond rol daar in die stront rond.*" (Translated: "Woofie the collie dog rolls around in the shit.")

Considering I once got an award for miming, I suppose I did this well.

It added a nasty perception of human nature, where it seemed that nothing escaped the intention to humiliate, and it evoked memories of my time in the army.

I cannot recall how often they harried us into performing these demeaning acts and few readers will appreciate the sense of indignity.

I didn't want to complain but the final straw occurred late one evening, when there was a knock at my door and, as I opened it, someone hurled a bucket of water into my room soaking most of my expensive books.

Perhaps I was homesick, but probably just frustrated by the harassment.

Something must have snapped.

Pining to return home, I called my dad from the phone at the end of the corridor.

I had resigned myself to the fact that I would abandon my plans to study medicine and return to the bank or even play in the Army Band.

I mean, what else could I do?

Looking back, the impulse was understandable.

(I might add that my second-oldest son did this 30 years later. After attending classes for a few weeks, he returned home from Pretoria University. How strange that I did not empathise with him.)

The following morning, I was throwing clothes haphazardly into a suitcase, when there was a loud pounding on the door and, as I opened it, a large man with ramrod-straight posture in a military uniform confronted me.

I recognised the booming voice.

"So, canon donkey, where the hell do you think you're going?"

It was Staff Parker from the Army Band!

My despondent parents, desperately looking for someone to reason with me, had contacted Staff Parker from the Army.

I started to explain that I was packing my bags to return home, but, before I could complete my sentence, he interjected: "No, my friend, you are coming with me. Ma and I will look after you."

He lifted my bags in one hand, draped an arm around

my shoulder and led me to his car.

He shoved my things unceremoniously into the boot of his green Citroen, and within an hour we'd arrived at his home in Voortrekkerhoogte (the houses of the South African Defence Force).

"Welcome Pietertjie," Ma Parker invited me into their home. She looked kind and fun-loving, and it tickled me that she called me Pietertjie, which is Afrikaans for little Peter.

Standing at her kitchen door in a floral apron with her three sons and a daughter at her side, she took my hand in hers and led me into the house.

It was a home where everyone seemed comfortable and happy.

I got to know a different Staff Sergeant Parker. He was a doting father of five with his eldest daughter already out of the home. He insisted that the kids address me as "uncle" – a sign of respect in the Afrikaner community for anyone older than you. I was only 20, and the eldest son, Francis, was a pimply faced 16-year-old, so it felt weird.

All the kids (Francis, Hennie, little Eric and Ronel) had to call me "Uncle Peter", but Ma always called me Pietertjie.

Their outside domestic servants' quarters became my room.

It had a single bed and a bookshelf with a toilet and shower and was actually very comfortable.

Living with the Parkers was one of the happiest times of my life and I suppose you could safely assume that if

it were not for them, I would never have completed my
medical degree.

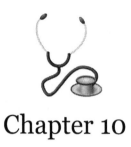

Chapter 10

Cat Skull

As one of my zoology projects I had to get a cat's skull to show the numerous foramina at its base, and someone suggested that I try the Pretoria SPCA.

To my horror, they offered me the entire head of a euthanised cat.

At first, I had reservations; then I thought, *Why not?*

I took it and, if you will excuse the pun, headed home.

But I needed to strip it of the flesh and hair.

So, stay with me on this. Since I'm rather squeamish, you might not believe the following story.

Ma Parker was not home, and I thought I could remove the flesh by cooking the head.

Looking around in Ma's kitchen I found the ideal vessel – a large pressure cooker.

I half filled it with water, popped the head into the pot and put it on the stove with the dial set to high.

As the cat's head steamed, the whole house filled with

the aroma of something cooking.

At around 4.30pm, Ma arrived from work, and called out, "My goodness, Pietertjie (her endearing name for me), what are you cooking?"

A grin spreading over my face, I tried to squirm my way out of the situation – momentarily considering telling her I was cooking a dish for some friends – then admitted what I was doing...

Nothing could mollify her, and the vivid recollection of that raving, screaming woman remains etched in my soggy brain to this day.

Serves me right!

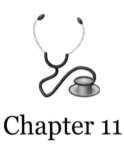

Chapter 11

You Need Guts To Get Through Second Year Medicine

If you've never heard The Seekers singing *I'll never find another you* and *The Carnival is Over*, then perhaps you can watch them now (check them on YouTube).

Go ahead – I'll wait. It will set the mood for 1967, the year in which I braced myself for the stress of second year – when one actually studies medical subjects.

The class of '67 was the first in the new BMW Gebou, a modern five-storey building with state-of-the-art facilities.

Medicine isn't rocket science. It may actually be easy, but the training, during which one's self-confidence nosedives, is arduous.

The   second-year   subjects,   physiology   (with

biochemistry) and anatomy (with histology), get expanded in a later year with pathology, microbiology and pharmacology.

Anatomy and histology describe the structure of the human body, and physiology and biochemistry the normal function.

Anatomy, the architecture of the human body, is the bedrock of medicine.

Pathology is the study of disease where the structure and function fail, and microbiology introduces the infective causes of disease.

It seems obvious that the curriculum was crafted to provide a foundation for the problem-solving skills needed by a doctor – information that will translate into the practice of medicine.

A sound grasp of these subjects separates even a highly experienced nurse or paramedic from a graduate doctor.

You can think of disease as three sides of a triangle labelled "biological", "physical" and "social", with the human organism in the centre comprising one's soma and psyche.

Although most clinicians might shudder at this over-simplification, I find it a nice way of thinking about it.

My first encounter with the anatomy dissection hall was a daunting experience.

We assembled in a spacious lecture room, where the head of the anatomy department, Prof. Tobie Muller, prepped us about respect for the deceased.

The *Ou manne* (students who were repeating the year) had spread the word to choose a male cadaver, the contention being that the layer of fat beneath the female skin became rancid, causing the body to smell.

I'm not sure how true this is.

After Tobie's lecture we traipsed downstairs through the heavy double doors to the hostile and bleak dissection hall.

The students trickled in, first with expressionless faces, then gawking at the sight of bodies lying in rows on cold metal gurneys.

The stench of formaldehyde that suffused the air overwhelmed my nostrils and the sight of the bodies wrapped in plastic and cloth was unnerving.

How weird that one then referred to the dead as cadavers and not bodies.

And how and when did *He* or *She* became *It*?

I teamed up with William Taylor, and we scurried around lifting drapes to see if the corpse underneath was that of a male or a female.

Students milled around calling out, "This one's mine!" and we had to move on to find an unclaimed body.

We settled for a large person who we reckoned was most likely a male, and "staked our claim".

I took a deep breath and, hands trembling, gingerly unwrapped the upper part to reveal a man in his mid-fifties.

Four of us shared a corpse; William and I worked on the cadaver's right.

Most students named their cadavers, and we christened ours Cassius – after Cassius Clay the world champion boxer, who later changed his name to Muhammad Ali.

Anatomy is indispensable to medical training, with cadaver dissection every day of the week.

I suspect that with so many subjects now clamouring for the students' attention, dissection might not receive as much training time as it did in those days. It's even possible that a virtual cadaver might someday replace actual dissection of a real person.

Every morning, following an anatomy lecture, we went to the smelly hall to dissect that part discussed in the lecture.

We found ourselves squeamish, scared and excited simultaneously.

It's an eerie experience to see a corpse so stark and one tried to detach oneself from the fact that this was once a living, breathing human being.

But I guess the allure of anatomy is that you get to see something that few are able to.

It's where the dead teach the living – a romance that's hard to deny.

At first, I pinched my nostrils and pressed my jacket collar against my nose, but not long afterwards I became blasé and relaxed, and even recall bringing a Coke and a *koeksuster* (Afrikaans confectionery) to the hall during dissection.

Dissection of a cadaver is like an archaeological excavation. To get to the deepest layers, one works from the top down. The process is anxiety-provoking and enthralling—a medical school initiation rite with almost religious overtones.

Most students respected the dead, but there were always a few "livelier" candidates.

One group behind me dissected blood vessels that had been injected with a coloured elastic substance (to make the arteries more visible) and flicked them across the room.

I often had a few such projectiles striking me on the back of my neck.

One embarrassing moment was when two guys crept up from behind and wrapped their cadaver's colon around my neck, just as the lecturer entered the hall!

Although it had little to do with me, since cadaver respect was taken very seriously, I was in a lot of trouble.

(So, you can say that it took *guts* to get through the second year.)

In December 1967, having passed second year, I accompanied my parents to Cape Town for the Christmas holidays.

It was a Sunday morning on the 3rd of December and, as we approached an intersection, my eye caught a billboard attached to the traffic light.

"Stop the car!" I called out, indicating to my dad to back up a few metres.

There, in thick black typeset, I read: SA PERFORMS WORLD'S FIRST HEART TRANSPLANT.

This was at a time when there were enormous objections to swapping body parts. Kidney transplantation had taken hold, but a heart! This was something extraordinary!

With my knowledge of cardiac physiology, I tried to figure out how this was possible. It wasn't just the anatomical and immunological aspects that intrigued me. I couldn't get my mind around the physiology of a heart beating without nervous connections. I don't know why, since I had spent weeks in the physiology laboratory demonstrating how a frog's heart could beat outside its chest, provided that you gave it the correct nutrients. We had studied the effect of infusing adrenalin and elements like calcium and potassium and had recorded the effect of the contractions using a revolving drum blackened with soot.

How the heart transplant had happened was that Denise Darvall and her mother had stepped out of a bakery and were crossing the road carrying a cake for Denise's dad's birthday, when they were struck down by a drunken driver. The mother was killed instantly and the 25-year-old Denise was seriously injured.

Denise was declared brain dead at Groote Schuur Hospital and her distraught father allowed the enterprising Prof. Christiaan Barnard to remove her heart and transplant it into the chest of Louis Washkansky.

The dramatic story of the world's first heart transplant makes exciting reading, so you can imagine how it beguiled a second-year medical student. Even Washkansky referred to himself as a new Frankenstein!

So, Barnard replaced Livingston as my hero.

I attended a lecture he delivered to the Pretoria medical faculty following his achievement. He had a curious accent, which I managed to emulate.

I got so good at performing a Chris Barnard impersonation that my colleagues Charles Niehaus and John Riley would repeatedly goad me into putting on a performance.

One of my favourite recollections was when Barnard explained death.

He said that previously they considered a person to be dead when he or she had ceased to breathe (a mirror was held in front of the person's mouth to see if it misted).

Later when it became evident that you could keep someone alive with ventilation, they assumed death when the heart stopped.

Electrical defibrillation and cardiac massage put an end to that notion!

Barnard never elaborated on the idea of brain death, but in his characteristically charming manner he exclaimed that a person is only dead, "when the doctor says he is dead."

He described the scenario where a deceased person is transported in an ambulance to the hospital ER and the casualty doctor gets into the back of the ambulance to examine the man.

When the doctor states: "This man is dead", then and only then is the man considered dead.

It was a humorous story but still profound. Death is a syndrome and the doctor makes the diagnosis based on the features of that syndrome.

I would entertain my friends with this story, telling it like Barnard did with his characteristic accent!

Once when we were holidaying at a hotel in Port St Johns, the barman was so enamoured by my stunt that he gave us a free meal!

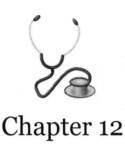

Chapter 12

Porter at Addington

A vacation job as a porter at the Old Addington Hospital in Durban gave me a taste of working with real patients.

The old building now squats in the looming shadow of the new 15-storey Addington Hospital, and both face the Indian Ocean with the most pristine beaches.

Old Addington was a drab cream-coloured three-storey colonial-style structure. It had a maze of passageways crammed with patients on trolleys. There was an internal courtyard with wards reached by lifts with old-fashioned ornamental, but efficient, iron-laced cage doors.

The highly polished cement floors had areas with fading linoleum, and large ceiling fans cooled the spacious wards, but I don't remember any air-conditioning.

The nurses' little hats projected an image of neatness and servitude, and their starched white uniforms spoke of institutional dignity.

I had been to Addington in 1958 when my dad, Paul and I had arrived in a taxi one afternoon to fetch my mom, who had just given birth to my sister Margaret. As we pulled up to the front entrance, I distinctly remember asking if she was a boy or a girl, and suggesting that, if she was a girl, "We could swap her for a boy!"

It was weird being back there and trying to navigate the hospital's mazy structure.

Since I was a medical student, management let me work as a porter in the theatre complex.

The matron was a solidly built woman in her late forties with jet black hair just visible under her cape.

Miss vR ruled the theatre with an iron fist, and she terrified me, but everyone respected her.

In those days they re-used latex gloves and one of my chores was to clean the bloodstained gloves. After cleaning, each glove was hung up to dry, turned inside out and again washed and hung up to dry, then turned again and hung up to dry.

I am sure this confused you as much as it rattled my brain writing it. (Like those typographic glyphs.)

Each glove was tested for holes and, if any were found, put aside for patching!

The gloves were sorted by size and side (left and right hand), put into a folded paper envelope and sterilised in an autoclave with a small packet of talcum powder placed in the upturned cuff.

This is a far cry from the disposables used these days.

My student loan, with a generous contribution from my dad, helped me to buy a light blue 1961 DKW junior, which, with its three-cylinder two-stroke motor, sounded like a coffee grinder as it went through the three-speed gearbox. The car gave me new independence, but my starter motor malfunctioned and I had to push to start it.

Mr Jacobs was an elderly man who operated the sterilising autoclave in the central sterilising department (CSD) and on hearing about my car problems he said that if I could slip the starter motor through to the theatre complex, he would repair it for me.

The following day, I parked alongside the theatre block, removed the motor, and with it wrapped in newspaper I trudged up the stairs and made my way through the theatre swing doors.

Matron vR sat at her desk facing the open door, and I had to pass her office with the grease-covered contraption.

I headed for the autoclave room and gingerly negotiated the terrain, then made a brisk dash past her door.

As I passed, I heard an ear-splitting shriek, "Mr Desmarais, what the hell have you got there?"

I retraced my steps, stumbled and, standing in her doorway, stammered that I was taking my motor to Mr Jacobs.

"Just get that bloody thing out of this theatre immediately!"

There was no opportunity to negotiate, and I bolted out through the swing doors clutching the broken motor.

I can't say I was popular with the matron after that.

On Monday mornings, visiting surgeons operated at Addington.

Some surgeons had the most uncanny names, to wit: Butcher (a surgeon), Bull (a gynaecologist), Hogg (a nose surgeon), Batchelor (a gynaecologist).

Imagine an electrician named Spark, or a plumber named Flush and you can understand my fascination with these names.

When the surgeon *du jour*, Nigel Butcher, discovered that the porter in his theatre was a second-year medical student, he turned to me and asked, "Well now, boy, would you like to scrub for the next case?"

I jumped at the offer to scrub, with the intern and me assisting the surgeon.

Nobody had taught me how to scrub and gown, so I watched the houseman and tried to emulate him.

He opened the taps with his elbows, so I also pushed the taps open with my arms. I copied him as he used his elbow to depress the dispenser and squirted liquid soap rubbing it into a lather between his palms. He scrubbed his nails, hands and forearms while keeping them in the air.

I mimicked his every move.

Suddenly, he turned and blurted out, "Stop looking at me. I don't have a clue how to scrub!"

(I later learnt that the more junior member of the surgical team – usually the intern – should never finish a scrub before the senior surgeon. This is a part of the hierarchy in medicine.)

While it was embarrassing to have to stand on a bench

alongside the operating table, I felt important donned in the green theatre gown, mask and cap.

Having just completed my first six months of dissection, I had a sound grasp of the anatomy of the chest and pectoral muscles so I could follow the mastectomy operation.

The surgeon removed the breast and – quite uncharacteristically for the demure Mr Butcher – tossed the severed organ towards me.

As I ducked, the organ struck the floor with a plod and a squelch!

There can't be many students who assisted at live surgery in their second year, least of all any who ever had a tit thrown at them.

What a baptism into surgery!

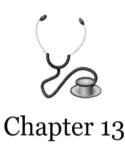

Chapter 13

The Quack

(Spoiler alert! This chapter is hardly amusing, but it may give you an idea of why I think most alternative medicine is a load of crock.)

Medicine evolved over the years from quackery to become a science – it's not completely there yet, but it does strive to be science-based.

So-called alternative medicine is when a discipline stubbornly refuses to embrace science.

And when doctors accede to an alternative remedy, they might accidentally give succour to the world of pseudoscience. How sad is that.

Although my mother treated our childhood illnesses with natural remedies, I wonder if any could be supported by science and how many were just based on hearsay or folklore.

We had friends in Durban whose son was a naturopath and herbalist, and I earned pocket money working in his practice during my mid-year vacation.

This Machiavellian prince called himself Dr Philip and his "Herbal Health Clinic" was behind Addington Hospital, strategically situated to attract patients on their way to the hospital.

Control of practitioners seemed less stringent than nowadays.

From the outside the clinic looked like a pharmacy with a window displaying promotional signs: "CURE YOUR ILLNESS THE NATURAL WAY" and "NATURE HAS THE CURE TO CANCER THAT YOUR DOCTOR DOES NOT TELL YOU ABOUT".

As you entered, there was a counter, with shelves containing rows of medicines in colourful containers behind the counter.

There were large gaps in the wall behind the bottles, allowing you to just see through, but the display was so busy, you could not see Dr Philip sitting in his office behind the wall. However, Dr Philip could see if some-one approached the entrance.

He had an imposing oak desk, scattered with health magazines and snapshots of his family. On a shelf behind him was a statuette of a Greek god with a large phallus and, on the wall to one side, posters of acupuncture points of the human body.

In my naivete, I assumed that Philip was medically qualified.

He used the title of "Dr" and displayed the certificate of a fake DOCTORATE OF HERBAL MEDICINE degree on one wall – a qualification supposedly conferred on him by the University of California.

But he had scant medical knowledge – his grasp, especially of anatomy and physiology, was so rudimentary as to be non-existent.

If by looking through the gaps in the wall he saw a customer entering the shop, he would step around to the front to serve them.

A little old lady once came in and asked for advice. She'd had cardiac failure diagnosed by the doctors at Addington Hospital and she showed him the bottles of medicine they had prescribed.

The labels read: Digitalis, Hydrochlorothiazide (a diuretic) and Slow-K (a potassium supplement).

Gripping the little bottles, he sneered: "Do you know how poisonous this is? More people have died from Digitalis than from the attack on Pearl Harbour!"

With his hand lightly on her shoulder, he appeared to show some concern. Then in an outlandish act of showmanship, he tossed the three little bottles into the wastepaper basket!

It was an act as unconscionable as it was cruel.

Unfazed, he then offered the hapless woman two jars of his "health-giving herbs".

"These will get you right within a few weeks" he said. "I normally charge R40 but since you've been so poorly treated by the medical establishment, I'll happily give them to you for R20."

Quite pleased, the woman left the clinic clutching the jars.

I wanted to say, "Wait a minute", but I never spoke

out, and it plagued me later. I wondered how many such victims may have died from pulmonary oedema alone in their room.

The herbs came in large wooden tea boxes and we would fill different bottles labelled for diverse ailments from the same box.

When I queried this, Dr Philip's reply was that herbal remedies were "ubiquitous" – his word for a panacea or cure-all.

I was sitting in his office when he said, "Peter watch this!"

He plucked out a long peashooter from under his desk, tore off a piece of newspaper and chewed the paper for a few seconds.

He asked me to hold up a few sheets of newspaper spread open about three metres in front of him and spat the chewed paper out of the pipe.

It shot out like a missile going right through at least three pages of the paper!

Then he said, "Now watch this," and stuck his peashooter through the gap in the wall pointing at the pavement in front.

A while later an elderly man ambled past the shop. Philip took aim with his pipe and spat out a projectile, which struck the guy below his chin.

He swung around, clutching at his bleeding neck.

Philip mouthed at me to keep quiet and dashed out to beckon the man in, offering to dress his wound.

"What the hell happened?" muttered the guy. There

was panic on his face.

Philip feigned concern. "Beats me, but objects sometimes fall from the sky from airplanes and kids also throw items at passers-by from apartment windows."

Then in another incredible act of audacity, Philip sold him a herbal remedy to prevent infection.

Dr Philip claimed to be the first person to put herbs into capsule form.

I sat with his parents, gathered around the radio when they broadcast it as breaking news on the 7pm newscast. It had supposedly followed ten years of intensive research.

Since I was there when he did it, it left me with a nagging feeling of complicity.

All he did was to get his assistant (the cleaner) to pour the herbal mixture into a sheet of cardboard rolled up in a cone (like you ice a cake). He placed empty gelatine capsules in holes on a strip of hardboard and filled each capsule with the herbs from the paper cone!

I doubt if the venture, from planning to preparing the paper cone, drilling the holes in the board and filling a thousand capsules, could have taken more than a few hours, let alone ten years.

And we scooped the same herbs from one tea box!

Since the amount now contained in each capsule was small, it gave Dr Philip an enormous profit margin.

Although this story has Darwinian undertones, it is an obvious and brutal fact that the gullible public needs protection from charlatans and money-grabbing psychopaths.

Purveyors of sham medicine prey on the desperate, especially before science has a solution to their illness. But patients are often lucky and get fooled into feeling better.

I imagine the polar ice caps will melt before we solve this dilemma, but it's worth re-emphasising that we need regulatory authorities to enforce science-based medicine!

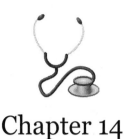

Chapter 14

Like Childbirth The Fourth Year Isn't Easy

Thank goodness gynaecology and obstetrics are subjects only taken in the fourth to sixth years. If introduced any sooner, I suspect there would be a mass exodus of students out of medical school.

Although giving birth is a natural process, it is never easy.

I have to this day an enduring horror of an obstetric mishap, mainly because of the following incident, which occurred at the end of my fourth year.

It was raining one evening in December and we had a full day of obstetric practicals at the Old Moederbond Hospital in Beatrix Street.

We were in the hospital tearoom huddled around a coffee table idly scanning through magazines when a large and somewhat officious-looking man in a dinner jacket with his tie undone and loose around his neck, appeared. His booming presence commanded attention.

In a thundering voice and pointing his finger at me he bellowed, "Doctor, you have just completed the third stage of a normal vaginal delivery, and your patient is bleeding. What do you do?"

I was unnerved by the challenge in his tone – he appeared to be talking to me and, since his stiff posture suggested that he was a lecturer or someone important, I felt obliged to answer the query about a postpartum haemorrhage (PPH).

"Well, I can rub up the uterus," I stammered.

On the wall opposite us was a washbasin, and he nudged the faucet handles open letting the water flow into the basin. "She's still bleeding," he said.

"Well, you can give Ergometrine by injection," I added.

He pushed the handles further apart, and more water flowed.

"She's still bleeding," pointing at the rushing water.

"We can put up a drip and give Oxytocin," I said.

He pushed the handles further, and the water flowed briskly.

"She's still bleeding," he snapped.

I scratched my head. In desperation I added, "Blood transfusion."

He pushed the handles further.

"Still bleeding," he growled.

The houseman prompted with more options: "Compressing the aorta, packing the uterus, tie off the uterine arteries," were his choices.

Then he pushed the tap handles fully open.

The water was flowing full force, striking the bottom of the basin and splashing onto the floor.

I was too busy gawking at the puddle to even notice his accidentally stepping into it.

I opened my mouth, but nothing came out.

There was an uncomfortable silence, then he said, "It's time to say: 'Doctor, call a doctor!'" and walked out.

"Who's that?" I asked the houseman.

He whispered, "It's Prof. Frans Geldenhuys, head of obstetrics and gynaecology."

That bleeding can be this dangerous after childbirth tells you all you need to know about the pitfalls of a normal delivery.

(They taught us in obstetrics that *it's only normal until it isn't.*)

It is not unheard of for such a patient to need up to 12 units of blood and still perish.

So, it's not surprising that I have an abiding fear of a PPH in particular, and of obstetrics in general.

On the other hand, I notice that – certainly in the developing world – hardly anyone has their babies delivered vaginally. Caesarean section has become the "go to" mode of delivery for indications that are often to say the least nebulous. C-sections are often performed apparently to ensure the best possible outcome.

The vagina will eventually have a one-way sign. It

will be an organ for entrance but not exit!

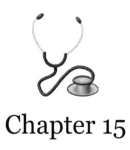

Chapter 15

Obstetrics Can Also Kill The Father

(This is the only chapter in this book of an event that I did not personally experience.)

O ur assistant professor of obstetrics stood waiting for the class to settle down.

On the table in front of him was an oblong ceramic porcelain basin with a small rag doll tucked into the cavity.

He explained that the interior represented the pregnant mother's uterus, and the oval opening at one end the birth canal.

The doll had a porcelain head and a body made from floppy material. One could place it in any obstetric position in the cavity (e.g. longitudinal vertex, breech or transverse).

Even the head position could vary, depending on

factors such as extension of the baby's neck.

Any student of obstetrics will understand this.

If that's you then, yeah!

As for the rest of you – sorry it would take half of this book to describe the positions and the mechanisms for delivery.

An interesting way of explaining the dynamics of labour is to consider the 3 Ps: Passenger, Power and Pathway (Pelvis).

The baby is the passenger who has to pass through the pelvic pathway, with the contractions providing the expulsive power.

The professor put the doll in a vertex position and with the head in occipito-posterior position (P.O.P), a position that does not allow the head to transverse the birth canal easily and, while obscuring the opening on top of the basin with his arm, he asked a student to demonstrate how he would carry out the delivery.

With his fingers in the opening at the one end, the student had to feel the position of the head.

He did the "vaginal exam" (PV) and said he would let the delivery go ahead naturally. The lecturer could then gently push the doll out while the student guided the head.

However, nothing happened, because the professor held tightly on to the doll.

After a few failed attempts, the student decided to apply forceps (so-called instrument delivery), and the professor handed the intrepid student a pair of Wrigley's forceps.

Then the fun began.

The student applied the forceps and tugged, expecting the "patient" to push during contractions.

But the professor held the doll and it wouldn't budge.

The student panicked and increased his force, but the professor held the doll firmly.

The class fixed their eyes on the porcelain mother and no one stirred while the minutes passed mercilessly away.

Suddenly the professor released his hold, and the doll shot out like a cannonball, flew across the room and slammed into the wall!

The Wrigley's forceps fell apart, the porcelain mother tumbled over onto the floor and broke into two pieces.

The bewildered student stared in disbelief and it seemed some time before he realised what had happened.

Unfazed, the professor stepped over the shattered model, picked up one blade of the forceps, and handing it to the student, bellowed, "Now sir, take this instrument and smash it over the father's head, and you will have successfully wiped out the whole family!"

You need to look no further for evidence that obstetrics can be disturbing.

With catastrophe constantly beckoning, it's no surprise that when I chose a speciality, obstetrics was not on my list...

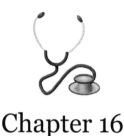

Chapter 16

Forensic Medicine – You Just Need A Body

The forensic medicine professor was a middle-aged man of medium build, who wore black-rimmed glasses with thick wavy lenses. His bushy moustache tightly twisted at the ends covered his top lip, and the only discernible sign of aging was his slightly greying black hair.

A permanently grim expression bedecked his features, and he looked like Sherlock Holmes, pacing stiffly back and forth with an unlit pipe clenched between his teeth.

All that was missing was a deerstalker cap and a cape. (A curved calabash pipe might also have added to the likeness.)

He was an oddball, and he mystified me.

In some odd way, his unusual name, Professor Haranimus van Praque Koch, seemed to suit his bent for forensics.

His lectures were profound, but his appearance and demeanour distracted me so much that I often failed to listen to what he was saying.

His moustached upper lip didn't help with communication and his rapid-fire way of talking made his lecture sound like a police report as he sucked on the pipe.

Bottom-line: I remember very little of what the man said.

I do, however, recall a lecture about potential injuries in a head-on motor vehicle collision. I craned my neck forward to watch him pacing from side to side, his arms folded behind his back and his jaw jutting out.

"Ladies and gentlemen, with a sudden deceleration, one can get an avulsion of the aorta, or one cannot get an avulsion of the aorta." A most fatuous comment if ever there was one.

If you weren't paying attention, you could easily have missed the second part of his sentence!

Forensic autopsies rely on a regular supply of material, but, with so many fatal motor vehicle accidents and murders in South Africa, there was no scarcity of victims.

One afternoon he entered the lecture room, leant over the lectern and, pointing the stem of his pipe at the class, the austere Haranimus growled, "Ladies and gentlemen, a student complained that there were no bodies at the mortuary yesterday."

He cleared his throat and continued: "What the hell

do you want me to do – go out and kill someone for you!"

Such remarks brought much-needed levity to his lectures.

Mind you, Haranimus failed to extinguish my interest in forensics, as you might gather from the following experience.

It was 1969, the year of Woodstock and my fourth year at medical school.

I had found a two-bedroom flat in Kotze Street, Pretoria, which I shared with two of my best friends, Smittie Steenkamp and Allan Visser.

Smittie invited me to spend a holiday on his farm in Karasburg in South West Africa (now Namibia) and I jumped at the offer.

Summer had just given way to autumn when we made the exciting and scenic two-day train journey from Pretoria down to De Aar and then back up through the Northern Cape to South West Africa.

I had the time of my life and have cherished the camaraderie for many years thereafter.

Students were partying on the train and it made for a rollicking ride with round-the-clock frivolity and togetherness.

Alcohol flowed freely and someone strummed the guitar to the tune of the Beatles' song *Ob-La-Di, Ob-La-Da*:

Ob-la-di ob-la-da life goes on, bra
La-la how their life goes on...

Ob-la-di ob-la-da life goes on, bra

La-la how their life goes on...

Karasburg station was just a railway siding with no platform. The train arrived in the early hours of the morning, and Smittie's dad drove us in his Mercedes along a seemingly endless stretch of narrow tarred road and finally along a twisting gravel road to pull up at the Steenkamp family farm about 30 km away.

Much of this land is arid, so it didn't surprise me to see wide-open expanses dotted with unglamorous dwarf shrubs and the weirdest plants eking out an existence in the desiccated landscape of South West Africa – arguably the driest country in sub-Saharan Africa.

The Karakul sheep here are desert sheep and survive on the sparse vegetation. Their pelts get marketed as the prestigious Swakara, but it marred my visit when I realised that they slaughter just-born Karakul lambs within a day of their birth.

It was something that was definitely not nice to watch.

With the declining demand for Swakara pelts, I imagine that this industry might not survive.

I visited the local hospital hoping they could use my medical student skills and Smittie arranged for me to spend a few days with the resident doctor, Paul Smith, who also had a private practice in the town.

But when I arrived at the hospital, I found the good man had gone on a three-week vacation, leaving the hospital – and indeed the whole town doctor-less.

The local pharmacist provided primary care with a

senior nursing sister running the hospital and it felt a bit unreal that I would be the only doctor at the hospital.

I got a kick out of running the outpatient clinic, suggesting treatment for minor ailments, and I recall impressing a nurse with my knowledge of dermatomycoses (fungal skin infections).

Dermatological terms are guaranteed to impress the layman and while we can name the affliction, in most cases we seem ignorant of the cause.

The sun had just risen one morning when an open truck pulled up outside the hospital. At the back was the body of a young African man covered with a sheet of canvas and the driver pointed out that the unhappy man had decided to end his life. They'd found him hanging from a tree.

We carried the shirtless and bare-footed body into the hospital casualty area and placed it on a metal gurney. It was deeply unsettling seeing the body with the thick mark around his neck and I could not stop myself from considering how abruptly and meaninglessly life can end.

He had swollen eyes with his conjunctivae injected with little red blood spots (petechiae). The fluid around his mouth was dry, and the rigor mortis suggested that he may have died many hours before.

I had an idea: since I had recently studied forensics, I suggested to the nurse that we should do an autopsy.

(You can decide whether this was out of courage or plain stupidity.)

We scoured the cupboards and found the requisite instruments lying haphazardly in a corner against a wall with some thick black gloves and a red plastic apron.

Eager to do my first unsupervised post-mortem (PM), I mentally revised the steps I had learnt in forensics as we wheeled the corpse into the little mortuary.

The body lay naked on a shiny stainless steel surface that reflected the harsh glow from an overhead theatre light and, just as I was about to begin, I heard a grating sound and, through the window, I saw a white truck pull up outside the mortuary.

Two uniformed policemen stepped out. One was a tall black constable and the other a wiry white man with a beard and frizzy grey hair. His hands and face were darkened by the sun and he had a two-pip officer's rank.

They entered the room and asked to speak to someone in charge.

Well – the senior sister was in charge, but I was arguably the doctor.

Someone had told them about the deceased and they had come to collect the body.

I stepped up. "But I need to do an autopsy before you take the body," I objected.

Then the Afrikaans-speaking officer retorted in very broken English, the vernacular of the area, "But jus why does you need to do it when we's know vat he died from – hanging himself," he said.

"Well, we still need to determine the cause of death," I insisted.

He stroked his goatee and frowned. "But we's know

it. He died 'cos he hanged himself."

"Yes, but how do we know that he was not killed in some other manner?" I pleaded with him.

"What other way...?" he sneered at me as though I had done something wrong.

"Well, he could have been shot or something..."

"Do it looks like he been shot?" said the officer, waving his arm over the corpse.

I raised my hand in a gesture of resistance. "No, but–" I began.

I got no further. In a flash, they grabbed the guy – the officer at the feet and the constable holding the head – and carried the body to their truck, where, with a disturbing clunk, they dropped it in the back.

Within minutes they had gone.

So that was South West African law in the '60s.

And I missed the opportunity to perform my forensic PM.

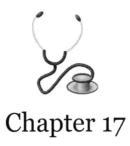

Chapter 17

1970 Sixth Year and the Lesson I never Learnt

On a stifling November day during my final year, I found myself sauntering along Schoeman Street in Pretoria. It was a dull moment and I was spacing out, with nothing better to do. (Quite unusual for a final year medical student.)

On the opposite side of the road, I spotted a car dealership and, gracing the showroom floor, was a beautiful yellow Alfa Romeo GT junior.

I crossed two lanes of stalled traffic to get a look through the reflective glass.

It was a drop-dead gorgeous car.

As I shielded my eyes to get a better view, the salesperson, a portly Afrikaans man in a beige safari suit, confronted me.

"You like it, hey?" he said, snuffing out his cigarette against a pot plant.

"It's beautiful."

"What do you do?"

"I'm a medical student."

"Really, what year?"

"Oh, in my final year," I remarked nonchalantly.

His eyebrows lifted. "Final year? Are you going to pass?"

"Pretty sure," I said confidently.

Suddenly his demeanour changed, and he addressed me as "doctor".

He opened the driver's door, "Come and sit inside, doctor."

It was sufficient encouragement.

I slid into the Alfa, ecstatically fondling the steering and was smitten by the plush interior with the black velvet seats.

Oh, sooo black.

The new-car smell aroused my senses and the ignition key seemed to beckon – "Turn me on. Oh, please turn me on."

He slanted a glance at me. "Do you know I can put you in this car today, doctor?"

It sounded too good to be true.

"That's impossible!" I blurted. "I haven't any money."

"Tut, tut, doctor. You don't need money. You can take it today and make your first repayment in February next year."

"Yeah, and what about a deposit, and the cost of licensing and registration?" I said rather awkwardly.

"No no, you need nothing – we organise a lease and

amortise the costs into the deal."

I had never heard of a lease and he pointed out that professional persons like me qualified for a lease.

I listened casually at first, then more attentively.

I liked the way he thought...

It was no longer a question of how, but when!

What a salesman.

A week later I drove out of the showroom with a spanking new Alfa Romeo sports car.

This dalliance with decadence did not sit well with the poor boy from Newcastle.

I paid the price for this extravagance; it was my first step into debt, from which it took almost a lifetime to recover.

I don't know how you can convince young people that expensive cars will, you know, lead to chronic pain in the wallet.

It almost sounds dumb now that I put it into words.

Buying a fancy car is like marrying a stripper. It's great at first, but you know it will end in tears.

For it is written:

Blessed are they who delay gratification and control their impulses – for they will inherit the wealth.

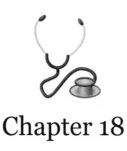

Chapter 18

Daspoort Policlinic – I Had To Bring It Up

It amazed me to see how many poor people lived in the Pretoria West region, distressed communities who could not afford private healthcare and had difficulty getting to the provincial hospitals for minor medical problems.

The faculty of medicine at the University of Pretoria used this as an opportunity to train students while offering a much-needed community service.

They commissioned an old house in Daspoort to use as a clinic.

There was a clinic every Friday night.

Second-year medical students did the immunisations and injections. Third-year students worked in the pharmacy, fourth-year students assisted the "doctor" and fifth-year students were the doctors!

A visiting GP supervised everything. The sixth-year

students were too busy to work in the clinic.

It was fun doing a stint at the clinic where the patients called you "doctor" and were genuinely grateful for the help.

When I started my fifth year, I tried not to miss Friday nights.

It was an eye-opener to see the spectrum of disease in the lower-income groups. Diseases that usually appear in old age are common in younger less privileged people. It seems a higher income really makes a difference.

A middle-aged, unkempt and morbidly obese woman attended the clinic most Fridays. She was scruffy, with hair tied back, layers of grime caking her skin and an offensive odour that filled one's nostrils.

I remember her small rigid toothless mouth, her smudged lipstick and her rasping breath.

She wore dirty blue sweatpants and her feet were in sockless homemade slippers, which I couldn't stop staring at.

She seldom smiled or spoke, and I cannot recall what her medical problem was, but I remember the halitosis and a stench that lodged in the back of my throat. (*Oh, where was Mother Theresa when you needed her?*)

It was, to put it mildly, a harrowing experience examining her.

There was no way this unkempt woman could have had a happy home life. Why she was like that was a mystery, but George Orwell makes this remark: "Poverty frees them from ordinary standards of behaviour."

When we saw her sitting in the waiting area (the

lounge of the old house) we would "draw lots" to decide who would examine her.

One Friday, I drew the short straw, so I had to see Mrs "Smelly".

She sat in front of me, her purse and coat clutched under one arm, and smiled as she related her problem of recurring abdominal pain.

Struggling to climb up to the examination, her balance teetered as she lifted herself, and I leant in to help.

Examining her was not a nice experience. Had she *ever* bathed or changed her clothes?

(Okay, that was a bit of an exaggeration. Forgive me, dear reader, for bringing this up, but it took all of me not to!)

I had an idea: I asked the students in the pharmacy to pour 400 ml of Savlon into a bottle and to label it "the solution – not to be taken". I then told her we needed to clear her body of "toxins". (This was nonsense of course.)

Instructions were to add two capsules to a hot bath and soak twice daily for 30 minutes.

The following Friday the tubby woman was sitting in the waiting room sporting a clean skirt and a pair of Nike sneakers.

I stifled a smile as she greeted me with her toothless grin, and everyone was amazed when I actually requested Tannie as my choice.

I held her hand and chuckled – she smelt like a lily!

Now more than 47 years later, I wonder if she is still bathing in Savlon!

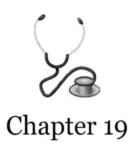

Chapter 19

Home Remedies – Do They Work If You Don't Grow?

Most medical schools have an annual student conference, and the medical faculty of the University of the Witwatersrand (Wits), in Johannesburg, held their 28th congress at the Wits medical school in May 1971 during our final year.

Professor Derksen, our chief of general surgery, addressed us in the circular tiered lecture room. He read a memo from Wits inviting a Pretoria student to present at the congress.

The invitation seemed virtuous, but I speculated that they had a perverse reason for choosing the topic: *home remedies.*

These so-called *Boererate* were used as alternative medicine by rural Afrikaners.

It was common knowledge that the Wits students fancied the TUKs students to be rural doctors.

Professor Derksen, a highly revered man in his early sixties, had a half-halo of grey-white hair framing his balding pate. He was kind-hearted, with a perpetual welcoming broad smile, and would entertain students with his down-to-earth approach to surgery.

His lectures, told with twinkling eyes, were humorous stories that would transport you to another place and time.

(Research confirms that we remember facts better if we're exposed to them in a story.)

Here is one that comes to mind.

It was a lecture about the five cardinal signs of inflammation, which the Roman, Celsus (no, not the Swede who blew hot and cold), described in his extant treatise *De Medicina* in about 5 BC.

Calo (warmth), *dolor* (pain), *tumor* (swelling) and *rubor* (redness and hyperaemia), to which someone later added *Functio laesa* (reduced function), made up the signs.

Derksen's eyes sparkled as he said: "So, one morning your neighbour leans over the fence and asks your mom if you could look at her gardener's painful knee. Since you are in your fourth year of medicine, and in your mother's eyes already a doctor, she asks you to pop over to give Mrs Jones an opinion.

With your brand-new stethoscope dangling conspicuously out of your lab coat pocket, you bend over to examine the leg.

You feel for any warmth, inquire about pain with movement; you see no redness, and the movements appear normal.

Then you stand up confidently and proclaim: 'I don't know what is wrong with the knee, but since it lacks Celsius' cardinal signs, there is no inflammation!'"

Derksen's eyes lit up as he told this story, emphasising the five signs with his outstretched fingers.

Anyway, turning back to my story:

He surveyed the class. "We want someone who speaks reasonable English to represent this class at the Wits conference."

I got full marks in a surgical exam, and Derksen had thereafter called me his "little surgeon", and his gaze fell on me.

"Tunguy, my little surgeon, I think you should go," he said.

Being called "little surgeon" sounded like a character from Snow White, but I overlooked this.

I can't say I was thrilled, but, if you recall that I grew up in a home where my mother used natural remedies, I was probably best qualified to give such a presentation!

There is an uncanny belief that anything natural is good for one's health, a virtue that resonates for nebulous reasons.

My take on this is that nature intended 2 of your 5

children to die and for you to perish by 50, so there's a constant battle for science and technology to outsmart nature!

And heaven forbid, do not decamp from your spot at the base of Mount Etna when that seismograph convulses. C'mon – volcanoes are natural.

But my mother had raised us on those *boererate*.

I waded through two thick black volumes in the municipal library and it surprised me to discover that there were about 2000 "remedies" recorded with the Zuid Afrikaanse Akademie vir Wetenskap en Kuns (South African Academy of Science and Art).

The texts described the craziest remedies imaginable. One could ease the bronchospasm of asthma by smoking pawpaw seeds in a pipe. Pumpkin pips helped rid one of intestinal worms and inhaling the burning hair of a cat could also break an attack of bronchospasm – to mention only a few.

Most of these remedies lacked rigorous testing but could have a modicum of scientific plausibility, which makes for a lively discussion. I think the burning cat's hair might release nitrates, which may help explain the smooth muscle relaxation.

Quacks who used pawpaw seeds for asthma knew that papaverine (an alkaloid of opium) relaxed visceral muscle spasm and assumed that it would also relieve the bronchospasm of asthma.

That it helped might be entirely serendipitous, though, because I doubt if pawpaw releases papaverine.

(It's just that in Afrikaans the name papaya sounds similar. The Spanish also call it papaya.)

I prepared my lecture with slides and an overhead projector, and for some comic relief – to displace my anxiety – I peppered it with humour.

When it was my turn, I faced the audience (remember that I am only five foot two inches tall) and, with sly jocularity, said: "Ladies and gentlemen, I *grew up* on home remedies," and – pointing to my short stature – I added, "As you can see, they don't work!"

The dean of the faculty, an elderly gentleman sitting at an arm's length from me, almost fell off his chair chuckling.

It was another occasion when to my surprise I received an award for practically nothing. This time, the Westdene prize for the best presentation at a student conference.

I still have these slides after 49 years!

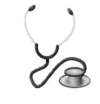

Chapter 20

Final Exams – It Depends

Oral examinations follow the written tests in medicine.

They are just a formality because the examiners already know whether the student has passed the written and practical examinations. It was a way of establishing how we reasoned and presented ourselves.

I had my final oral examination in internal medicine at the medical school.

My examiners were the bulldog-faced Professor Zaidy, a laconic man of fierce intelligence, who rarely smiled, and an external professor from the Wits medical school, whom I did not recognise.

One never knows whether one is properly prepared. Waiting, I fumbled with my notes, which I then stuffed into my lab coat pocket.

I felt small and vulnerable sitting in front of the professors.

Zaidy smiled and seemed not to know how to put me at ease.

The other professor, whom I was not even looking at asked, "Could you describe the features of cardiac failure?"

"Well, that depends," I said.

"Depends on what?" he asked.

"Are you referring to acute or chronic cardiac failure?"

"I would like you to describe the features of chronic congestive cardiac failure," he began again.

"That depends," I retorted, averting my eyes from his glare.

"What does it depend on now?" came his irritated reply.

"Are you talking about small babies or adults?"

"I am referring to adults with congestive cardiac failure!" he practically shouted.

"Well, that also depends," I said.

"What the hell does it depend on now?" He sounded angry.

"Well, sir, the features depend on the cause. It is different in a person with hypertension compared to someone with Beri-Beri."

"Beri what?!" he blurted and turned to face Professor Zaidy, who smiled and nodded.

"Just go [sic]..." said the visiting professor.

I got a distinction pass in medicine and the gold medal.

(Sorry about tooting my own horn, but, as with my Orpheus Award, I wish I could proudly say that I deserved it.)

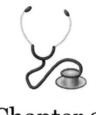

Chapter 21

Intern – The Allure Of Addington

I had to choose where to do my internship year.

Well, I actually only needed to decide whether I preferred to do a gruelling year as a houseman or sail around the Greek Isles…

I wanted to remain at the Academic Hospital, where – provided I enrolled for a master's degree in clinical pharmacology – I would get a post as a clinical trials physician.

A ten-line letter from the hospital informed me in very technical Afrikaans that I had secured a six-month internship in the department of medicine, followed by six months in general surgery.

The paragraph about my accommodation was curt and official, and read: "Please present yourself at Room 102, where you will be allocated appropriate accommodation."

My friend Alan Visser (with whom I shared accommodation during my clinical student years) received an enticing three-page response.

This was the gist of it:

Dear Dr VISSER,

Welcome to Addington Hospital, Durban!

We are a 720-bed hospital with the following amenities:

And the letter described the comforts and attractions of the hospital, the Durban beachfront and Durban as a tourist centre!

I read his letter with pangs of jealousy.

I *envisioned a suite in the Addington doctors' quarters with a coffee-making machine, masseuses with hot rocks and a Hi-Fi.* (We didn't have TV in South Africa until the late seventies.)

After six years of slogging, the allure of Addington Hospital was too much, and I followed Alan to Durban – a decision I never regretted.

(Admittedly a year on the Greek Isles would have been better.)

A few days later I composed a letter to the Chamber of Mines thanking them for the bursary that had enabled me to complete my studies.

I wasn't sure who to address my letter to, or if anyone in authority would read or even acknowledge it, so I wrote a polite but brief letter (recalling Colin Powell's quotation).

My letter:

Bursary Dept.,

Chamber of Mines,
Hollard Street,
Johannesburg.
Dear Sir,
I would like to thank you for helping me realise my dream.
Yours,
Gideon Peter Tunguy-Desmarais.
(I swear the letter was as short as this.)

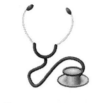

Chapter 22

Medical House Job at Addington Hospital

Although internship is harsh, and one spends the time trying to avoid a mental or physical break-down, I just loved my time at Addington, which, as I've mentioned in previous chapters, was a modern 15-storey, 720-bed hospital in a superb setting. Why, it had the Indian Ocean as its front lawn!

It was exceedingly well equipped, and I felt privileged to work there.

As I explained earlier, I had been to the old Addington Hospital in 1958, before they had built the new building. This was the drab three-storey Victorian structure where my Dad, Paul and I had arrived by taxi one afternoon to fetch my mom and Margaret, my newborn sister, and where I'd asked whether the baby was a boy or a girl, and then remarked that if she was a girl, "We could swap her for a boy!" It was also where I had worked as a porter in my second year of studying medicine. (I wrote more about my experiences in the old hospital in Chapter 12.)

The new building was south of the old and boasted a smart and modern nurses' home. I later learnt that the jaw-dropping Addington Nurses' Home – not mentioned in the letter to Alan – was the main appeal for young housemen. There was certainly nothing surprising about this.

(Overheard in Doctors' Quarters (DQ): "So many nubile (libidinous?) maidens, so little time!")

It was Sunday of the first week in January. The vibrations of my alarm jarred me out of my peaceful sleep.

I heaved myself out of bed, wiped the sleep from my eyes and opened the blinds to an overcast sky. Although exhausted from my move from Pretoria to Durban, my adrenalin would not let me relax.

The day before, I was a student. Now – rather abruptly – I was a real doctor in the real world and would have to make serious decisions.

My first thought was to suss out the wards.

The rain was bucketing down as I ran across from DQ to the hospital foyer, where I bumped into Kallie Schilz, the only guy from my final-year class who was shorter than me.

He was waiting for the elevator in a crisp white lab coat with one hand on his hip and a black umbrella at his side.

He greeted me with, "So how's the little prick?"

Just then the public address system crackled: "Calling Dr Schilz, calling Dr Schilz – for Ward 3A."

Kallie pushed out his chest and smirked: "That's me!"

He seemed so proud to be addressed as "Doctor".

That evening I took the time to explore the hospital and to familiarise myself with as much of it as possible.

The wards were strikingly modern and spotlessly clean, as if dirt had been outlawed, and my shoes squeaked on the shiny fluorescent-lit linoleum floors. Everything, from the theatre complex to the admin block, was superb, and one had a good feeling on entering any part of the hospital.

The following morning, dressed in grey flannel longs, a crisp white button-down shirt, with slim tie and a University of Pretoria blazer, I gathered my courage and presented myself at Ward 12A – female medical ward.

Sister Sinclair, a short plump woman with curly brown hair and gaps between her front teeth, was the ward charge sister. She was pencilling notes on a patient's chart.

I approached her and, although I said nothing, she appeared irritated by the intrusion.

She looked up, "Can I help you?"

"I'm here to see Dr Good."

"Dr Good is busy with a ward round. You'll have to wait," she said.

"Uh, okay," I mumbled, "Where should I wait?"

I was standing in the passage, so I expected her to invite me into the office.

"Well, you could wait where you are," she said, with an air of reluctance.

So, with my back to the wall, I stood – surviving the disapproving glances of the porters and the uniformed nurses passing by.

I stood for two hours!

Just after 10am, Dr Christopher Good, a tall thin man with angular features and a receding hairline, strode down the passage flanked by a retinue of medical officers, interns and nurses.

He almost passed me but hesitated when Sinclair chimed in: "Dr Good, this young lad is waiting to see you."

"Yes, my man?" said Good in a very British accent.

I wanted to beat my hands on the ground, but mumbled, "I am Dr Desmarais, your new intern. They told me to present myself to you today." I felt awkward using the title for the first time.

"*Doctor*! ...Desmarais!" the sister exclaimed. "I thought you were a schoolboy! You never said you were a doctor!"

I battled to maintain my composure, but Christopher Good seemed amused.

I could see the twinkle in his eye as he welcomed me to his department with an outstretched hand.

Despite this experience, I was fired up to be Dr Good's houseman.

They do not expect interns to know anything.

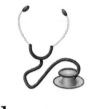

Chapter 23

Ward 12A, Bloviation and Rambling On

My first ward round with the pompous Dr Good was memorable.

I don't want to dismantle the idyllic image of doctors doing ward rounds in the *Grey's Anatomy* TV series, but it is anything but romantic.

Ward round teams would consist of an intern or resident, a registrar (usually a senior houseman at Addington) a consultant and, of course, the sister with a few nurses.

Clad in white coats, the doctors and nurses would gather around a patient's bed with the intern responsible presenting the history:

"This is Mrs S, a 70-year-old female from Durban, who was born in Benoni but spent the last 10 years in Natal. She presents with..."

The intern would then describe the presenting

symptoms, medical history and findings of the clinical examination.

Unless someone needed to contribute to the history, the presenting interns would not normally be interrupted.

It was my turn to present.

I folded my arms and cleared my throat. "Mrs A is a..."

I stammered but carried on, "a 60-year-old..."

Dr Good interrupted, "Goofy," he said. "Do you know what inspired Walt Disney to create that character?"

"Err, no sir," I said, baffled by the interruption.

He seemed to have a fascination for Walt Disney and proceeded with a lengthy interpretation of Disney's choice of characters.

I don't think I listened to much of it.

When he stopped, I continued, "She presented with a complaint of..."

"Bambi," Dr Good resumed his Disneyland segue. "This character was inspired by..."

He continued for half an hour or so, while we stood shuffling from one foot to the next.

Christopher Good appeared to thrive on an eager audience and I swear the ward round with his Disney fixation continued like this.

Why he did so I'll never know, but it was an extraordinary challenge to one's patience.

I imagine each new intake of housemen gave him another captive audience.

Someone told me they call this bloviation. (One

wonders why?)

Ward rounds were a four-hour-long ritual that warped space and time and the downside was that it left little time for clinical work the rest of the morning.

But despite this, my intern training in internal medicine was superb.

Christopher Good died many years later from some form of encephalopathy.

During my time with him, I admired his knowledge and abilities and regarded him as a good (no pun intended!) clinician with a most retentive mind.

He exuded an air of uprightness and respect and, as you can tell, I had huge respect for him. (A well-named fellow.)

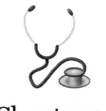

Chapter 24

Intern Stress and Plasmapheresis

Interns are brutally overworked, doing long hours, juggling commitments and having to cope with sleep deprivation.

My phone would ring at ungodly hours like 1.50am. "Sorry to bother you, doctor. Are you sleeping?"

No, I lie on the operating table every evening – I wouldn't dream of sleeping!

By the end of my first week, I knew that I just wanted to sleep.

It's a "survival of the fittest" experience – one is bleeped for one emergency after another – enough to make Sisyphus throw up his arms.

Sometimes I worked all day, all night and most of the next day – not once stepping outside to see if it was sunny, overcast or raining.

Each new day picked up where the last one ended. I

was so tired following a night session that I could hardly stand on a ward round and would stay upright by holding on to a drip stand.

Sometimes I'd sleep on the ward – or more likely fall into a coma!

(The nurses once set me up with a mattress in a room next to the nursing station reserved for counselling family members.)

I'm convinced that internship is the last bastion of slavery. (There aren't many ways to escape this other than perhaps to move to Canada, above the 49th parallel.)

Fatigue greatly enhances the risk of error and harm, and while as students we'd spent a third of our life studying, we were hopelessly unprepared for the daunting task ahead of us.

Managing situations where one doesn't have a freaking clue is no fun.

All humans make mistakes, but when a doctor makes a mistake, they shame him in court, on TV and online (that lives on forever). *One suffers the agony of harming someone else – unintentionally – for the rest of one's life.*

It was grim, but the prevailing attitude was that one had to grin and bear it.

That was simply how things were.

It was not always the long hours or the load of responsibility that got to me, but the frustrations really knocked the stuffing out of me.

How sad that sometimes the only way to protect one-self was to stop caring.

But if one did stop caring part of one might die and never come back.

By the end of the year, most interns would have lost the verve and enthusiasm with which they started the year.

Mrs Visagie was just a small example of such frustra-tion. She was a thin 60-year-old lady, dark hair gathered in a bun. She had an autoimmune problem and a blood dyscrasia. Her exact diagnosis escapes me, but I had to take blood (venesection) five or six or even more times a day and send a unit to the blood bank. There they sepa-rated the plasma from the cells, filtered out unwanted antibodies and added back the cells. This "cleaned blood" was transfused back into her, a process known as plasmapheresis.

She winced as I approached her with the wide-bore needle and venesection kit, and we soon ran out of veins.

I tried her arms, her legs and her neck and became increasingly disheartened.

I attempted (to little avail) to cheer her up with bad jokes during the IV placement but, from the outset, I had an inkling that what I was doing could be an exer-cise in futility.

Late one afternoon while attending to Mrs Visagie I noticed Dr Gregg, the visiting haematologist, who was there to see a private patient.

Gregg was an amiable middle-aged man with an accent to match his obviously Irish surname.

He was completing notes and never saw me battling with the hapless lady, but he smiled and dragged his face upward when I entered.

I mentioned to him about the exhausting plasmapheresis and he responded saying that haematologists did not think it was of any value.

I put my head in my hands. Wow – talk about deflation! Was I torturing poor Mrs Visagie for no good reason?

Now I know why people self-medicate!

It was the proverbial last straw. Frustrated and clutching the blood bags, I stomped up to Dr Good's office and did something I thought I would never do.

I didn't knock or wait to be invited in. I pushed his door open and deposited myself in front of a smiling Dr Good.

Without flinching, I slammed the blood-filled plastic bags down on his desk amongst the clutter of books and papers, and, as corny as it sounds, asked why we were bothering with plasmapheresis when Dr Gregg considered it worthless.

(I think sleep deprivation may have caused my churlish behaviour.)

Dr Good, the quintessential gentleman, silenced me with a reassuring, "Now, now, young Desmarais..."

There was an awkward moment, then seeing me so frazzled, he changed tack and promptly organised for me to take a week's leave...

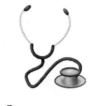

Chapter 25

The Big Prick and Let her!

As a student in my fourth year, I had done my psychiatric training at Westkoppies. It was considered one of the world's biggest psychiatric hospitals, where nurses moved from ward to ward on bicycles. Although I enjoyed the training, I felt useless handling psychiatric and psychological cases.

So, you can imagine my mood one Friday night just before Christmas when I admitted a young woman who had overdosed to Ward 12A at Addington. She was a stunningly beautiful 20-year-old with long blonde hair and amber eyes. They did a stomach washout in the ER before admitting her to my ward for observation and management.

The young lady settled in and I sent a request for a psychiatry consultation.

I completed the form:

"For attention: Psychiatry Department.

"Dr Good presents his compliments and requests your help with managing this case."

I described the patient and the problem.

On the Sunday morning I was sitting in the duty office enjoying the bright sunlight shining in through the windows on the opposite side of the passage. There was a rap on the open door, and I looked up to see a middle-aged man in a beige safari suit.

He waved a sheet of paper. "I'm Dr van der Merwe, the psychiatrist on call. Where is the girl who wants to kill herself?" He pressed his forefinger against his nose and lips.

I stood up mostly out of respect and pointed to the general ward, but he intimated that it would be better if we brought her to a private room along the passage.

So the patient, barefoot and wrapped loosely in a blanket, followed the doctor to the room.

In my naivete, I wondered what a psychiatrist and a wannabe suicide patient would discuss.

Would the discussion be about why she had found the prospect of the life ahead more than she could bear?

I sat there twisting my lower lip from side to side with my thumb and forefinger.

It came as something of a surprise that, barely 15 minutes later, the door opened and Dr van der Merwe emerged with an impassive expression.

He slammed the form on my desk and said: "Let her!"

And then he walked out.

I sat back and reflected quietly on what I had just experienced.

How infuriating it was that he must have concluded that her suicide attempt was just attention-seeking behaviour. Or had something else transpired?

While you may have agreed with Van der Merwe's made-for-TV moment, I thought he was a real prick...

A month later, I heard that the prickly doctor had killed himself.

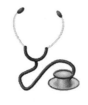

Chapter 26

Dr D and My Heart Lecture

One morning, I was again sitting in the warm sunlight of the nursing station, completing blood request forms, when a tall, rail-thin and slightly balding man, dressed in a beige safari suit, poked his head through the open door.

Those days psychiatrists and admin workers mostly wore those beige safari suits. (I wish I knew what trend spurred this.)

He looked important.

"Are you in charge?" he asked.

"I am the medical intern," I responded. "Can I help you?"

He regarded me suspiciously: "Yes, can you tell me about Mrs Papenfus?"

His tone was condescending.

I attempted a smile, "Why do you need to know?"

He waved a brown folio. "I have this letter from the family, who are concerned, and I need to reply."

He pulled out a sheet of paper.

I studied him and thought, *These admin guys – I suppose I had better give him some info.*

"We admitted Mrs Papenfus with dyspnoea and cough, and a chest X-ray suggested pulmonary TB. However, when our investigations proved non-contributory, we considered lymphangitis carcinomatosis – that means a malignant spread to the lungs," I explained.

His tone changed. "Yes, yes, but why was she admitted acutely?" Some cynicism had crept into his voice.

Then I made an awkward effort to explain her pathophysiology.

"Well," I said, staring at his short pants and socks, "the lung is like a big sponge that takes in air, but also blood from the heart. If the right side of the heart – which pumps the blood *to* the lungs – can't push the blood through the lungs because they are less resilient or scarred, the blood pools back in the vessels much like a blocked stream and a dam. The hydrostatic pressure of the liquid – the blood – in the vessels then forces fluid from the blood vessels into the tissues around the vessels, which then swell. We call this oedema, and these are the features of congestive cardiac failure," I said, emphasising the last three words of my sentence and gesticulating the actions of a heart and a pump.

I followed the explanation up with some expressiveness: "It's like flooding in your own fluid."

The surly man raised his eyebrows, his frown

deepened and he looked quizzically at me.

Then he blinked his eyes, gave a long sigh and stormed off with the file in his hand.

I drew in a lungful of air and turned to the sister at the desk behind me.

"Who is that man?" I asked.

"Oh, that's Dr D, the medical superintendent!" came the reply.

Eeek! Somebody later told me he was a Grinch and that I might have taught him something...

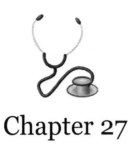

Chapter 27

Mrs Forbes Ablaze

There is one incident that stands out in my mind more than any other.

One morning on a ward round with Dr Good, we stopped at Mrs Forbes, who was in the second bed on the left. She was a thin elderly woman, with her dark brown hair a mess of curls and dark rings under her eyes. I had admitted her via the outpatient department with fever and a cardiac murmur.

I presented her to Dr Good.

"What's the likely diagnosis?" he asked in his pompous tone.

I pointed out that, unless there was another likely diagnosis, one should consider subacute bacterial endocarditis (SBE) in any patient who had a fever with a cardiac murmur. (These days they refer to this as "bacterial endocarditis", where bacteria in the bloodstream infect the heart valves.)

"Precisely," nodded Dr Good. "And what are you

going to do?"

"A blood culture, sir," I said, much to his delight.

"Right," said Good and, turning to the rest of the medical team, added in a spirited voice, "Young Desmarais here will do a blood culture and enlighten us," and we moved on to the next bed.

After the round, I asked a young nurse to assist me with the culture. I wanted her to ignite a few drops of methylated spirits (dripped on to the rubber cover of the lid of a blood culture bottle) and I would inject the patient's blood into the bottle.

Dear reader, I'd like to describe in some detail how my Pretoria teachers taught me to do this (far different from how it is done today).

The aim is to avoid contamination as you transfer blood to the sterile culture bottle.

So, they taught us to do a full scrub – like prepping for surgery. One dons a gown, mask, cap and sterile gloves. A nurse cleans the forearm with an antiseptic solution and applies a Baumanometer cuff to the patient's upper arm (blood pressure or BP apparatus.)

She covers the arm with sterile drapes and the operator, using a sterile syringe taken from a sterile wrapping, draws blood from the cubital vein, a vessel near the elbow.

Then the nurse squeezes the tiny amount of meths (highly flammable) onto the rubber seal of the lid and lights it with a match. The doctor withdraws the syringe and drives the needle through the flame into the bottle (through the rubber lid) and squirts the blood into the bottle.

This was sterility at its best!

It was unimaginable that a bug could have crept from anywhere into the bottle, and, if they cultured an organism, it could only have come from the patient's bloodstream.

Dressed in my theatre gown and brandishing the needle and syringe, I approached Mrs Forbes. I must have looked like one of those doctors who handle Ebola cases.

Anxious and scared, she fidgeted with her sheet, but I reassured her that it was just another way of drawing blood.

She clenched her fist as I drew the blood and, out of the corner of my eye, I noticed the nurse pouring the "meths" from a wide-mouthed bottle onto cotton wool. Glug-glug.

I had a nagging feeling that something wasn't right.

She squeezed the cotton wool, drenching the bottle with the meths and, as she was about to strike the match, I realised that there was indeed a problem.

"Noooo!!" I blurted out, under my mask.

Toooo late.

As she struck the match, there was a blinding flash and an explosive whoosh.

A ball of fire drifted into the air like a burning meteorite!

It was surreal...

Now, I only discovered later that the fluid the nurse was pouring onto the cotton wool (chug chug style) was not methylated spirits at all! It was ether! Flammable. Explosive. Volatile.

Highly!

This explained the "fireball" – the flammable vapour was burning in the air.

A blazing ball hovered in mid-air.

(I wonder if you can imagine "fire hanging in the air".)

The fireball floated down and landed on the trolley with the dressings, cleaning fluid and syringe wrapping paper.

Flames leapt down the sides of the blood culture bottle and almost everything on the trolley caught fire – including the paper wrapper, which wafted into the air and landed on the patient's bed!

I yelled, "Kill it, kill it."

"With what?" stammered the nurse.

"With this!" I shouted and grabbed a dish of pink cleaning solution from the trolley and dashed it onto the bed.

It was Hibitane spirits – also flammable!

It was like the feeling one has reaching for an escaped balloon.

With another dramatic "whoosh" the flames leapt up to the ceiling, and some licked at the curtains around the bed.

(Pandemonium reigned, and the royal children, Mayhem and Bedlam, frolicked about.)

People rushed in from everywhere.

Someone ran in with a fire extinguisher and sprayed thick white foam all over, leaving the ward looking like a blizzard had blown through and dumped snow everywhere.

(While not funny it was reminiscent of the Peter Sellers classic movie, *The Party*.)

Mrs Forbes, with terror in her face, was yelling obscenities...

(I could have sworn that she was crying, "Help – I'm being cremated!" but perhaps I've imagined this over the years.)

She signed the RHT (refuse hospital treatment) form that afternoon and left.

I have a vivid recollection of pushing the blackened and charred trolley down the passage, my hair singed...

So, lesson learnt.

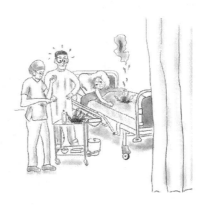

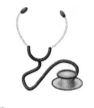

Chapter 28

Hayden and the Defibrillator

The women in medical Ward 12A were mostly elderly.

Mrs vR, having suffered a cardiac event two days previously, was hooked to one of the three monitors at Addington Hospital.

I loved the monitors, which nowadays are ubiquitous, and it intrigued me to see a patient's ECG come to life on the oscilloscope with the reassuring familiarity of a normal BP and pulse rate. This gave a beep, signifying acoustic proof that life hadn't given up on the person.

Transcutaneous oxygen saturation recording – nowadays also commonplace – was unheard of at that time.

Mrs vR was the mother of a senior theatre matron at Addington Hospital, the same matron who five years earlier had chased me out of the old Addington theatre block.

I cringed when she visited her mother, hoping that she wouldn't recognise me as the porter with the broken starter motor.

One morning I was standing in the ward and glanced in Mrs vR's direction to see her suddenly clutch her chest. I noticed the cardiac tracing change from an apparent "sinus" rhythm to the zig-zag pattern of ventricular fibrillation, effectively cardiac arrest.

It was just as well I was there.

Ashen, she slumped back, and I rushed to her bed, calling for help.

She was pulseless and not breathing – the features of cardiac arrest.

Managing this as a young intern is dramatic and exciting (these days I would be happy to shirk it).

The management is ABC – Airway, Breathing, Cardiac massage.

We sprang into action and, within seconds, there was a frenzy of activity. Getting the patient flat on the floor is better, but since there's a risk of skull fracture pulling someone down, we kept her on the bed and began external cardiac massage (hands compressing the chest), with mouth-to-mouth ventilation.

I could feel ribs cracking with the compressions – five to each breath.

A nurse rushed up with an AMBU[1]; we bagged[2] Mrs vR and someone set up a second iv line.

In between compressions, I shot in an ampoule of adrenaline, not even stopping to think if it was appropriate.

The quick-thinking nurse attached the AMBU to the wall oxygen and turned up the flow.

The oscilloscope confirmed the diagnosis of Ventricular Fibrillation (VF) and, since there was a built-in defibrillator, conditions were ideal for resuscitation.

Since most readers will not be familiar with external cardiac defibrillation, here is the rundown.

When you're ready to activate the current, you signal to the team helping with the ventilation and chest massage to stand aside. Then, with the paddles in your outstretched hands on the patient's chest, you stand as far from the bed as possible and press the buttons to deliver about 400 joules.

There's nothing scarier than the split second before you push the buttons. (Being shocked *out* of normal cardiac rhythm is no picnic.)

I instructed the nurse to stop bagging her and held the paddles on Mrs vR's bare chest.

Just as I was about to press the buttons, I sensed a

---

[1] AMBU = the proprietary name Ambu, is a manual resuscitator or "self-inflating bag". It is hand-held and is used to provide positive pressure ventilation to patients who are not breathing.

[2] Bagging someone is medical slang for ventilating a patient with an AMBU bag.

commotion near the entrance to the ward with a man yelling.

Someone had called Dr Hayden R, the anaesthetic registrar.

He was a short and stocky Welshman with a mop of flaming red hair, an irascible personality and a temper, with the obligatory harried nature in tow.

I associated him with unpredictable buffoonery, and I was willing to bet ten bucks he would not last long as an ICU medic.

He sprinted in, frantically waving his arms, and on seeing the monitor tracing, called out, "Ventricular fibrillation, ventricular fibrillation!"

Not wanting to miss out on the action, he tried to shove me aside as he lurched forward to the patient. He hadn't noticed that I had already placed the paddles on the lady's chest, nor did he hear me shouting, "Clear the bed."

It was too late. I pressed the buttons as he grabbed Mrs vR's arm!

There was a vicious ZAPPP... Mrs vR's body shuddered and fell back onto the bed, and Hayden flew across the room with a wild flailing of his arms, landing on his butt a few metres away.

He landed under a wash-hand basin and slumped forward looking dazed.

I noticed that he had his right hand on his opposite pulse, which in retrospect judging by the smirk on his face could have been an act to impress us.

He hauled himself up and stumbled forward

muttering obscenities as he staggered to a nearby bed where he bent over and rested.

We had successfully defibrillated Mrs vR, who was in sinus rhythm and breathing.

She regained consciousness and happily made a complete recovery.

On her discharge, she thanked me with a packet of *koeksusters*.

Every few weeks thereafter, a parcel of *koeksusters* arrived with a note stating: "Thanks again."

As a coda to this story...A few months later the pastry sweets stopped arriving and I heard that she had passed away peacefully at home.

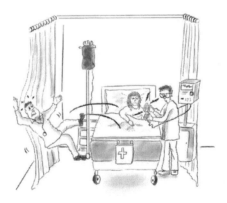

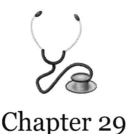

Chapter 29

Oh No – Have you Killed her?

Medical interns often see gastrointestinal bleeds caused by painkillers in elderly people. I am not sure what one can do about this because it happens despite education about the effect of these drugs on the stomach.

Why this advice is ignored so often is a question worth considering.

GP powders were a popular over-the-counter (OTC) preparation that contained the nephrotoxic (kidney damaging) phenacetin, with aspirin and caffeine.

Some years later, the phenacetin was removed, and the product only contained aspirin and caffeine, with the subtle suggestion that it was more effective! Yet brand loyalists continued to use and endorse the product.

When it became apparent that little old ladies were

damaging their insides imbibing the stuff, the company secretly changed the formula to paracetamol and caffeine.

Nobody seemed any the wiser, but at least it was a safer concoction.

It never ceased to amaze me to see how the formula changed over the years.

On one occasion it was just paracetamol.

Nowadays it is a blend of paracetamol, aspirin and caffeine, yet, unsurprisingly, the fervour for the brand has persisted.

Hopefully, consumers might these days be better informed, but I have my doubts.

During my fourth year of study, I got a vacation job unpacking cartons in the hospital dispensary.

I recall boxes of a stronger painkiller – Codis – with a sign on the box that read: "NEW CODIS NOW WITH PHENACETIN."

Scarcely a year later, the boxes arrived with a red sticker attached: "NEW CODIS, NOW WITHOUT PHENACETIN!"

If you'll excuse the pun, what makes this rather hard to swallow is that we have always known that phenacetin is toxic to one's kidneys, yet it was an included ingredient.

The mind boggles...

I was on emergency intake when we admitted Mrs AH with a massive haematemesis and melaena (vomiting blood and passing blood per rectum). She was an 80-year-old diabetic woman and had been brought in by her niece after she'd collapsed at home.

The ER staff had resuscitated her after she had vomited an enormous amount of bright red blood.

With her haemoglobin level at 6, I transfused whole blood, set up nasogastric suction and administered oxygen.

Dr Good, contemplating her management, stood at the bottom of the bed rubbing his chin with his thumb and forefinger as he often did.

He palpated her abdomen, did a rectal examination and, straightening himself, said, in his posh English accent, "We'll do a gastroscopy."

To the best of my knowledge, Christopher Good was the only resident gastroenterologist, and at that time they seldom did gastroscopies.

The scope showed multiple massive gastric erosions – something that those days had a heartbreakingly poor prognosis.

It is common for reclusive old ladies to survive on a deficient diet of tea and Marie biscuits while consuming inordinate numbers of analgesic medicines that contain aspirin (such as those headache powders). When one combines this with an assortment of anti-inflammatory drugs, there is an immeasurable chance of something bad happening.

Mrs AH was no exception to this.

Like many of her age with chronic joint pains from

degenerative osteoarthritis, she often took anti-inflammatory medicines, which included indomethacin and oxyphenbutazone (two popular medicines at the time).

So, Mrs AH was supplementing her prescribed medicines with aspirin and – to add insult to injury – also the headache powders.

Since I can guarantee you that this concoction will eat away at one's stomach lining, she might just as well have swallowed big bang drain cleaner!

There were no proton-pump inhibitors (PPIs) such as omeprazole, and a histamine antagonist (H2 blocker) such as Tagamet was seldom used.

Tagamet (cimetidine) was outrageously expensive. I recall having a sample of five tablets in my wallet and, if anyone asked me for money, I would show them my strip of Tagamet!

We gave Mrs AH Mist.magnesium trisilicate via the nasogastric tube (just an antacid), with intravenous fluids and blood.

Surgery remained her only option. (These days a PPI might have saved her life.)

I sent a request for a surgical opinion and while I wasn't there when the surgeon saw her, I later read his report. He concurred with the diagnosis but indicated that her age and general condition "precluded any surgical heroics".

This meant that they had, in effect, given up on the poor lady.

If you want perspective in life, you need to study medicine.

I had spent the week agonising about a decent sound system with speakers and an amplifier in my room and here was a poor lady with her life screwed.

I stood at the foot of her bed, a pang in my heart.

Dr Good popped in and stood alongside me.

"What more can we do?" I asked, grasping for words.

There was an awkward silence.

"Well, young man, there comes a time when you need to realise that there are limitations – in all probability, she will die."

Die! In my ward. Just from a little stomach bleed – he must be crazy!

I was stunned!

All she needed was a few bags of blood.

When Good left the ward, I had a plan. I told the sister that we would "be pulling out all the stops" and I decided to turn that corner of the ward into a mini ICU.

I wrapped a BP cuff around an arm, set up a second iv line, attached ECG leads to her chest and connected it to one of our cardiac monitors.

The ECG chimed but quickly returned to normal.

I inserted a nasal cannula to deliver oxygen, passed a bladder catheter and sent arterial blood in a dish with ice for an ASTRUP (blood gases).

She was on the oxygen and 15-minute observations.

Then I ordered more blood.

We now had two drips delivering blood to the hapless lady, and I piggybacked fluid with added Ephedrine.

A while later, the nurse called to say that Mrs AH's BP had dropped to 60/40.

I asked for an inflatable cuff that gets wrapped around the blood bag (like a BP cuff) to let the blood run faster into the vein – something used frequently in obstetrics.

This turned out to be a smart move and, with more blood running, the BP rose again.

However, it was only temporarily successful. The rise didn't last, and the BP dropped. 110...100...90...80...70 with a corresponding thready pulse.

We were squeezing blood into the hapless lady, but probably could not keep up with what was leaking out, and my mood sank an octave.

I looked for another cuff for the other bag of blood but could not find one.

Standing on a small bench to reach the bag high on a drip stand, and with my hands firmly clasped around it, I squeezed hard while the nurse monitored the BP.

I squeezed harder and harder, pouring fluids and pressors into what was probably a bottomless pit of hypotension.

With each squeeze the blood flowed faster.
Then suddenly the bag popped!

Blood squirted in all directions, striking the screen around the bed and dripping onto the floor!

A small stream of bright red blood flowed between the beds and down the centre of the ward.

I staggered backwards off the bench, pushing the curtain aside and with blood dripping from my arms, face and glasses.

As I groped my way between the beds, aiming for the duty room, the lady in the bed opposite sat bolt upright and seeing my blood-spattered face exclaimed, "Oh my god, you've killed her!"

Now you know how unsupervised interns spend their time.

It saddened me that Mrs AH did not have a more dignified death – she passed away a few hours after this incident.

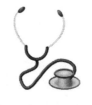

Chapter 30

Malaria – The Boyfriend And The Bike

All doctors need a lesson in humility and good medical praxis, which is to listen to a patient. They call it *taking a good history*.

But patients also need to know how to present their symptoms to a doctor.

It's called *providing a good history*.

During one's training, the incorrect use of medical terms by patients seldom gets emphasised.

Since very few patients have done that seven-year vocab course, there's no need to use a misleading medical term.

Imagine that you felt dizzy, and you told your doctor you had "vertigo". Guess what? If the doctor was pushed for time, he could enter your complaint as "vertigo" and, unless he applied himself, you could fall down the diagnostic algorithm of vertigo.

(Happens a lot with vertigo – if you'll excuse the pun.)

Vertigo is not a disease, it is a symptom, but it is a specific symptom pertaining to the vestibular system.

So, while all vertigo is dizziness, not all (probably very little) dizziness is vertigo, if you get my drift.

So, you might wonder why I make such a fuss about the distinction.

Well, I'll tell you.

One evening, a beautiful 20-year-old acutely ill girl came to the casualty department (ER).

She was feverish and told the doctor she had "flu".

It was late in the evening and the weary casualty officer, probably with a heavy workload, sneered at the late evening presentation of "flu".

"My boyfriend can only bring me in the evening with his motorbike, (sic)" she said.

I don't know if the doctor examined her, but he red-penned: "Came at 9pm – boyfriend can only bring her in the evenings with his motorbike!"

He gave symptomatic medication and sent her home to rest.

She returned the following evening.

This casualty officer again scolded her for presenting late in the evening with "flu" and again she alluded to the motorcycle.

The insouciant doctor drew a circle around the text "boyfriend can only bring her in the evenings with his motorbike!"

Happily, he made no other contemptuous remarks but added an antibiotic to her treatment.

The following evening, she presented yet again with her "flu-like illness" and a kindly and compassionate old GP (Dr Duncan), who was doing emergency casualty sessions, saw her.

"Why do you always show up in the evenings?" he asked, and again she mentioned the boyfriend and the bike.

"Well, this emergency room is for emergencies," he said, "but I'll get the medical houseman to look at you."

I was on call that evening and had been for the past two days.

Now, conscientious housemen ask pertinent questions (and boring things like your family history, your hobbies, pets, travel history and so forth), but they do examine patients well.

Most of my ward patients were geriatrics, so despite my 50-hour shift, you can imagine my enthusiasm when called to see this case.

I drew back the curtain. "What's the problem?" I asked, my heart pounding.

She wore a flimsy halter top and her long blonde hair fell over her shoulders.

Her makeup outlined her eyes, accentuating her pallor, and she appeared weary.

She brushed the hair away from her eyes. "I have a splitting headache and ache all over." Her voice was almost a whisper.

My cheeks warmed as I started my usual litany of

questions. "Are you normally healthy? Do you take any drugs?" On and on.

Then pausing, I looked at the notes.

In bold letters and circled in red were the censorious words: HER BOYFRIEND CAN ONLY BRING HER IN THE EVENINGS WITH HIS MOTORBIKE!

"What's this about your boyfriend and the motorbike?" I asked.

She dug around in a makeup bag for a headband and brush, then took a long breath, "Well, I have to come at night when my boyfriend is free and can bring me with his bike."

I realise it sounds dumb, but it was awkward chatting to this gorgeous blonde and, reflecting on it, I probably patronised her: "Aren't you nervous of motorcycles?"

She sat upright and didn't blink.

"Not really. We went to Mozambique by motorbike last week."

I put down the pen and rubbed my hand across the back of my neck.

"Mozambique? Did you take malaria prophylaxis?"

"No."

"Well, how do you know you don't have malaria?"

She leant back and a single line of a frown showed on her forehead. "How should I know? I'm not a doctor."

"So, who said you had flu?"

"I told the doctor I had flu."

"As you said, you're not a doctor, so how do you know it's flu?" – me exasperated, she weary.

Well, it didn't seem like the flu. No sore throat, no

cough and no known contact with flu.

(The diagnosis was probably lazy casualty doctor syndrome.)

But it's disconcerting that many people express any illness as flu.

She used "flu" as her presenting symptom!

She squirmed when I pushed against the right upper quadrant of her abdomen but there were no other clues at the examination.

There was a moderate pyrexia and a rapid pulse.

I wrapped a Baumanometer cuff around her upper arm and drew some blood, requesting a full blood count and malaria studies.

An hour later the lab tech phoned to report the ring forms of Plasmodium falciparum malaria.

My Swedish-trained registrar, the impossible-not-to-like Dr John Brock-Utne, had never encountered the disease.

John exuded an air of restless energy and spoke with the inflection of his native country. His face lit up and he chortled enthusiastically when I mentioned the diagnosis.

He examined the girl, agreed with the findings and asked about treatment. Since I had just completed my training, the dose of Chloroquine was fresh in my mind (500 mg stat, 500 mg after 6 hours; then 500 mg daily for 3 days).

But the wards had no stock and the dispensary opened only the next day.

At breakfast, I felt a tap on my shoulder and a gentle slap against the back of my head.

It was the relentlessly upbeat John, cheerfully whistling John Philip Sousa's signature tune: *The Stars and Stripes Forever.*

"Hurry up. We gonna treat our little malaria patient," he said, rubbing his hands.

"John, cut me some slack. She's just going to swallow pills!" I responded.

With his hand on my shoulder, we strolled off like a team to the hospital pharmacy.

I stood at the Addington Hospital dispensary drumming my fingers against the counter, but the pharmacist thought I was a bothersome jerk and refused to give the drug without the card.

We headed back to the ward, where the charge nurse sneered, "The cards get processed at 11am. Why can't she wait until then?"

I was at medical outpatients' later that morning when my pager buzzed with the message that my patient had collapsed while helping the tea lady hand out refreshments. They had alerted the ICU staff (and probably our friend Hayden,) and admitted her with suspected cerebral malaria.

I sprinted all the way to the ICU taking the three flights of stairs and, out of breath, I burst into the ward.

It was a moment of futility seeing her lying there and

wondering what more I could have done.

She was unconscious, intubated and on ventilation.

The next morning, I called in at the ICU – my patient had died about an hour earlier.

I don't know why her death upset me as much as it did, but I recall crumbling against the passage wall unable to breathe through my tears. The ache was indescribable.

Then I straightened my scrubs and went back to work.

The lesson is clear: take a good history and provide a good history, using the lay terms we all know.

And have a healthy respect for malaria. Since it can be fatal, it calls for prompt diagnosis and treatment.

Almost a million people die every year in Africa from this disease.

This killer may turn up after hours and on a motorbike. Disease doesn't care.

As a coda to this story:

The internet didn't exist when this event happened. These days more and more patients use it for health information.

I'm not saying that patients should not consult the internet.

However, one needs to depend on high-quality websites and research using peer-reviewed articles and sticking to reputable institutions (such as Mayo, Johns Hopkins, NIH and CDC).

In this way you can educate yourself, which is a good

thing.

Any doctor that doesn't want an educated patient is a fool.

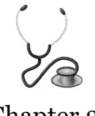

Chapter 31

The Cabbage Patch

I enjoyed my six months in medical Ward 12A, savouring any calm moments and cherishing the many experiences.

Interns would occasionally slip away during the day for a dip in the sea, but, being the nerd that I was, I seldom went to the beach during working hours.

There was an arrangement with the ward sister that if you were needed, she would hang a white towel out of a window for a few minutes.

On the only time that I took a splash in the Indian Ocean, I was in trouble. I wore glasses and had to scramble onto the beach every 20 minutes and put them on to see the ward windows. I left the water three times, retrieved my glasses and squinted up at the building, but saw no towel.

When I returned to the hospital about an hour later, I got reprimanded by the registrar for not being around when they needed me.

The sister had hung out a white towel but, without my glasses, I never saw it!

The female medical ward had mostly elderly patients, with the odd young person. I calculated the average age of an inpatient to be 78.

One would have thought that working with elderly people would be lousy, but the old ladies were beguiling and "grew on one".

Seeing the world through the eyes of the four demented and very confused patients in our four-bed annex was especially comical.

One morning the sister and I entered the ward and Mrs P, the old lady nearest the window, greeted me with, "Good morning, Captain. Where are we today?"

The views of the Indian Ocean were spectacular and, on sunny days, one could spot many ships and the occasional white sail of a yacht.

I glanced out the window and deadpanned.

"Well, Mrs P, we seem to have passed the Straits of Gibraltar," I said.

She waved her age-spotted hand with gnarled fingers towards the window. "Oh yes, I recognise the coastline!"

We all thought it was funny – and perhaps it was.

But, far from suffering demented anguish, this old duck was on a world cruise!

That's priceless.

I recall asking another: "Good morning Mrs S. How is your accommodation?"

"Well, I like the view, but the furnishing is a bit

sparse. Mind you, I shan't be doing any decorating."

It was entertaining and a point of grateful amusement.

The tycoon worried about the economy and stressed by his ulcerous marriage versus Mrs P sunning herself on the cruiser. Ask yourself...

I felt sad to leave 12A, where it pleased me to feel that I brought some sunshine into someone's life.

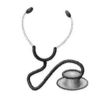

Chapter 32

Bloodletting – Even These Days

Bloodletting was a practice performed by surgeons in antiquity until about the 18th century – long before medicine evolved into a science.

(I guess it's important to recognise that modern medicine evolved from quackery into a science. Alternative medicine is to my mind a stubborn movement that refuses to embrace this.)

It was thought that one had to "balance the body Humours" to cure a disease and doctors did bloodletting with distressing ease and compulsion, often with consequences that ended badly.

I doubt if present-day quacks still do bloodletting but venesection for polycythaemia (where excess red blood cells are removed) is a scientifically justified procedure.

I was on medical call at Addington Hospital one evening when the ward sister, Joan Wild, reported that Mr

Gilder was battling to breathe. In his late sixties, Mr Gilder had been admitted that morning with cardiorespiratory problems and hypertension. He needed his BP controlled and his cardiac status assessed.

There were watery sacs beneath his eyes, which had bleary whites and red rims. The nurses had propped him up in the bed (high fowlers), because lying down aggravated his breathing (orthopnoea) but he was gasping despite receiving supplemental oxygen.

His pulse was rapid, and I noticed the ECG done on admission showed marked left ventricular strain.

The orthopnoea, tachycardia and noisy breathing were features of left heart failure (LHF) with pulmonary oedema (what the layman calls "Water in the lung").

They used Furosemide – a then recently introduced intravenous diuretic with IV theophylline and morphine in such situations. (I doubt if these days any of this, other than the diuretic, is used in LVF[3].)

As there was no Furosemide in stock, the sister went to search other wards for some (nowadays Furosemide is generally available anywhere) and, becoming impatient, I searched the cupboards.

I discovered a blood "giving set", which seemed to be ideal equipment to remove some blood from Mr Gilder. I reckoned it might bring him out of his pulmonary oedema by diminishing the load on his heart.

I couldn't assemble the set and, becoming frustrated, I tied a rubber catheter around Mr Gilder's upper arm,

---

[3]   LVF = Left Ventricular Failure

extended his forearm and neatly incised a distended vein.

The procedure was as simple as it could be, and dark red blood gushed out of his arm into a dish on the floor.

An astonished Sr Wild returned to find her patient with his arm dangling over the side of the bed and blood streaming into the bowl, but breathing normally.

It was something she would probably remember forever.

I allowed about a litre of blood to escape.

While certainly unorthodox, Mr Gilder's respiration improved by leaps and bounds as the blood left his body.

I am often tormented by the image of Mr Gilder with blood streaming down his arm, which in hindsight was a crazy thing to do. I mean, who renders a patient anaemic in the face of cardiac disease?

It's not quite textbook.

The following day they transferred Gilder to the high care ward, and I learnt that he left the hospital in good spirits and with his illness well under control.

I don't think Christopher Good knew about the bloodletting, because after I'd completed my internship in general medicine, he honoured me with a fantastic reference.

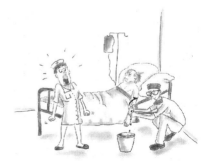

But one cannot rest on one's laurels.

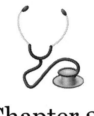

Chapter 33

First Surgical House Job - A Tinge Of Red

Training to be a surgeon is a graded process. One starts by observing surgeries, and later one practises to become an expert in assisting at the operation.

As a student, the senior or consultant asks you to perform the easier parts and you progress to more difficult parts – baby steps – eventually towards the full surgery.

Later you do the op with minimal supervision and then on your own with no help. That's when you get that indescribable feeling of being a surgeon.

Until then, you were just following instructions.

When you perform your first procedure, you have internalised your knowledge and your hand moves without your mind getting too technical about it.

Alan White was in charge of surgery, and I was glad to

do my first surgical house job under him.

White seemed to like me and called me "Petrushka" (his idea of a Russian version of Peter). From the outset, he ragged me about my interest in pharmacology, and claimed that the only medicine he believed in was iron – in the form of a steel blade!

I think deep down he admired anybody who had a knowledge of drugs and confided that Norman Sapeika, his erstwhile professor of pharmacology at the University of Cape Town and author of their textbook on pharmacology, had killed any interest and understanding he had regarding the subject.

In the surgical hierarchy, the chief of surgery is thought of as God and, in some respects, Alan White fitted this mould. He once yelled at an insubordinate intern: "Who do you think you are? Jesus Christ?"

The intern shot back, "No sir, just his houseman."

But underneath the white coat was a real person and an outstanding surgeon.

On my first day, I had to assist a visiting surgeon, Mr Roy Wise, with a vagotomy and pyloroplasty in theatre 2.

I scrambled up to the theatre block and was delayed looking for the change rooms, then struggled to find the theatre clothes, caps, boots and so on.

Getting dressed took some time because every theatre scrub top fell over my shoulders!

I stashed my belongings in a locker, stumbled out and gawked at the scribble chalked on a large green board in the passage.

They call it "The Slate".

My eye ran down the list...Wise...OT 2...Mr Watson...Pyloroplasty...

It was 7.35am when I stepped into theatre 2, aware of the beeping of monitors and the din of the ventilator bellows, and encountered a surgical team around a patient with his abdomen opened.

The surgeon was a thin man with features hidden behind his mask.

He turned and sneered: "Who are you?"

"I am Dr Peter Desmarais, the new house surgeon."

The bark of his voice surprised me. "Doctor Peter Desmarais, I put knife to skin at 7.30," he said without looking up. Then: "Do you read me?"

(When I wrote these lines 45 years later, I saw the retired Mr Wise sauntering down the passage at Entabeni Hospital on his way to consult with a neurosurgeon about his own extradural hematoma. We chatted, and I reminded him of the above, but he vehemently denied that he had ever said those words! My opinion is that he had become more genial over the years.[4])

Some weeks into my training, I admitted a young girl to 2A with suspected appendicitis. She presented with right lower abdominal pain and a bloated feeling. I pushed down over the right iliac fossa and she winced when I suddenly let go (so-called rebound tenderness).

---

[4] Roy Wise passed away peacefully in 2018

They teach one that the appendix sits at the pinnacle of intra-abdominal calamities.

And the dictum was: "The sun should never set on an acute appendix."

Roy examined my patient in the ward and ordered a stat appendicectomy.

He was sipping his tea in the theatre tearoom. "Are you keen to do the appendix?" he asked.

I was ecstatic – my first appendicectomy as a house surgeon!

"Well, tell Dr Communis you will do the case. He can assist you."

It was great that Communis, the much-liked surgical registrar, would be there to hold my hand.

He nodded and smiled when I asked him.

I bounced down the hallway, like Baloo humming *The bare necessities,* and slipped into an elevator, where – aware that no one could see me – I practised tying surgical knots on the metal barrier around the inside of the lift.

Back in the OT, the patient seemed to be at our mercy, asleep, intubated, naked and draped.

Anaesthesia is actually not sleep. It's something deeper.

A scrub sister stood alongside with an enormous and bizarre array of surgical instruments on a mayo stand.

Dr Ruben performed the anaesthetic, and I stared at the Boyles' machine. My eyes followed the black piping from the machine to the patient's endotracheal tube, and I stood for some time looking at the equipment, then at the sleeping patient.

The slip-shlop sound of the ventilator filled the room.

"Well, come on, boy. Get scrubbing," Communis interrupted my thoughts.

I scrubbed vigorously, dried myself and stepped into the sterile gown held open by the nurse, getting her to tie the strings from behind. The gloves were far too big for me, and I asked for a smaller size.

"What size do you take, doctor?" asked a nurse, but, realising that I did not know, she handed me a size 7.

With gloved hands held upright, I took my place alongside the draped patient.

I swallowed and something churned in my stomach.

Over my six years of study, I had often thought of this moment with dopamine-filled anticipation.

Suddenly six young nurses in theatre scrubs shuffled into the theatre in single file and stood against the opposite wall.

Unsettled I asked: "Who are these people?"

"Some students come to watch their first appendectomy," said their minder.

I craned my neck to get a better view of the nurses.

"But why has it got to be *now*? With *my* first appendicectomy!"

Dr Communis chimed, "Just relax...concentrate on

the op."

The scrub sister slapped a scalpel into my hand. I marked out McBurney's point and did the classical appendicectomy incision.

Blood oozed out. Communis swabbed and then sucked with a large metal Yankauer, which made a slurping noise, and I heard the electrocautery buzz as he quelled the bleeding.

I burrowed through the abdominal wall muscles and opened the peritoneum (the shiny membrane lining the abdominal cavity).

It's exciting to see the intra-abdominal organs (a lot better than the frogs I had operated on as a schoolboy).

I extracted a loop of small bowel looking for the appendix and pushed it back, pulled out more small bowel and replaced it. I did this three or four more times.

Then I followed the colonic taenia to where the appendix should be, but could not find it.

It seemed a lot harder than I thought it would be.

There was no time for small talk and beads of sweat rolled off my forehead.

The nurses were giggling, as they watched this little surgeon – the focus of all eyes – standing on a bench looking for the appendix which he could not find!

With an audience the pressure to succeed becomes enormous.

Communis took over and pointed out that the appendix was "retrocaecal" (where the tip of the appendix hides behind the caecum).

With his help and my pride cut to the quick, I completed the operation.

But the humility of the experience remains.

(I tell you, there was a tinge of red in that theatre on that day.)

Well, who is that unfortunate? One's first operation – a difficult operation – and a stadium of giggling nurses watching. Really?

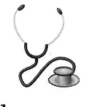

Chapter 34

Breast Abscess

A few weeks into my surgical training, I was asked to do a drainage of a breast abscess under general anaesthesia (GA).

I scrubbed and was ready at the operating table, but it surprised me to see the lady fully draped, but wide awake.

The anaesthetist was a lady from Croatia and told me to go ahead.

"But she's still awake," I protested.

In a broken accent, she explained that she was using neurolept anaesthesia (Ketamine) – something we almost never used in South Africa at the time.

There's a certain amount of fear and trepidation that comes with sticking a knife into a conscious person.

"Don't panic," I told myself, panicking.

Then I stuck the scalpel into the breast.

With that, the patient started singing: "Jesus wants me for a sunbeam, a sunbeam. A sunbeam..."

It was unnerving doing the whole op with the patient singing!

The funniest part was that after the op, as she was being wheeled down the passage, you could still hear her singing, "Jesus wants me for a sunbeam!"

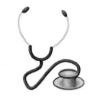

Chapter 35

Trapped in the Toilet

We were busy with a kidney op when I was bleeped to re-site a ward patient's drip that had "tissued".

It was early evening, and the 14th floor ward sent a nurse to hurry me on.

The surgeon, Mr Gray, said that the scrub sister could assist while I left to do the drip.

"Just get back soon because we'll be starting the next case," he barked.

Dressed in surgical scrubs, I headed for the 14th floor, re-sited the drip and took the elevator back to the theatre on the 3rd floor.

However, I pushed the wrong button and got out on the fourth floor.

"Damn," I cussed, and scurried down the steps to the third floor.

As I reached the stairwell, I heard someone crying: "Help! Please help me."

I stuck my head around the corner to hear the voice coming from the staff toilet on that floor.

I rattled the doorknob. "Hello, can I help? Who's in here?"

"Oh, please help me, I can't open this door. I've been here for almost an hour." It was the frantic voice of a woman.

"Who are you?"

"Mrs du Preez, I was visiting my husband and needed the loo. The door won't open."

Looking around, I sighed.

"I know this toilet; the door often sticks. You push and I'll turn the handle," I said.

"It won't open," she said.

"Okay, I'll push and you turn."

Nothing happened.

"Okay, I'll pull while you turn the knob."

Still nothing happened.

"I'm sorry, I can't help. I'm a houseman and I'm busy in theatre."

"Oh please, please don't leave me. I must get out."

I racked my brain for inspiration. Behind me, across the passage, was a dressing-room, and I scoured it for a tool. I found a metal tongue depressor, which I took to the door and wedged in the gap between the frame and the latch.

I don't have a clue how it happened, but, to my surprise, the door popped open.

Mrs du Preez stuck her head around from behind the door and rewarded me with the widest grin. "Oh, thank you, thank you! It was awful trapped in here."

Rather than letting the poor woman out and leaving, silly me wanted to prove a point.

"There is no reason you couldn't open the door; the sea air just causes locks to rust and stick," I added peevishly.

Then I did a crazy thing.

I edged past the lady, stepped inside the toilet and clicked the door closed while Mrs du Preez retreated against the toilet bowl.

As I turned the handle I said, "This is how it locks, and this is how it opens."

Whoops...the door wouldn't open!

I stumbled over the humongous Mrs du Preez's leg as she perched herself uncomfortably and unnaturally on the edge of the toilet.

I glanced sheepishly at her and my aggressive posture changed to self-pity.

(Looking back, I can only imagine the awkward scene: the two of us trapped in the toilet. There was me – in theatre scrubs – with this large lady squashed against the loo.)

"Don't worry. We'll get out," I tried to appear confident as I bashed my fists against the door.

After a while, there were footsteps and two nurses stopped to ask what was happening.

"Please help, it's Dr Desmarais and I'm trapped in the toilet with..." (I turned to Mrs du Preez) "What did you say your name was?"

"Du Preez," she mumbled.

"Mrs du Preez," I completed my sentence.

"But why are you in the toilet with a lady?"

"Never mind – it's a long story. Just help. There's a metal spatula on the floor in front of you. Wedge it between the lock and the frame and the door should open."

I heard grating sounds while they fumbled with the lock, but nothing happened.

I offered more suggestions, but nothing worked.

They passed the metal spatula through the Louvre vents low down in the door and I tried the spatula from my side.

The door would not open.

Moments later, a security guard arrived, and we repeated the conversation we'd had with the nurses.

"Dr Desmarais...Mrs du Preez...But why are you in there with her?"

Unable to open the door with the spatula, the guard left and returned a while later with a colleague and some tools.

They removed the outer part of the lock and passed a screwdriver through a gap in the Louvre part for me to dismantle the lock from the inside. This left a round hole about three inches in diameter and I peeped through the hole!

But the door would not open.

They removed the screws holding the Louvre frame and passed the screwdriver through a gap, and I pried the Louvre frame open from my side.

We now had a 500 mm x 300 mm opening where the Louvre was (at floor level).

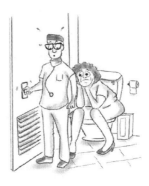

It was just big enough for me to squirm out.

I wriggled out on my knees and, glancing backwards, I saw the rotund Mrs du Preez's big head peering through.

"What about me?" she pleaded.

"Oh, you're too fat!" was my cutting rejoinder as I slunk away. (Only joking – although this was my thought.)

I took the steps two-at-a-time to the third-floor theatre, where Norman Gray was battling without an assistant.

"Where the hell have you been?" he blurted out.

I think I answered with: "You will never believe me..."

To this day, I don't know when or how Mrs du Preez got out.

The real absurdity of this is: Why did I get into that toilet?

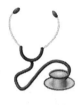

Chapter 36

Addington Fishing Trip

My internship ended on the 31st of December 1972, the day they formed the Addington Hospital fishing team.

Our first excursion was a deep-sea fishing trip.

It was a rather unfair competition since I was the angler with the largest tally to my name – probably a catch of about 250 *tons of fish* as will be clear in a moment.

The team members were me, three guys who had qualified with me in Pretoria (Derek van Deventer, Len Vermaak and Richard Venniker), Mike Grant, Tony Hamilton, and two honorary members, whose names elude me.

Everyone was up at 4.30am waiting outside DQ, but Derek had to shout from the parking lot to get me up.

The noise awoke a lot of doctors trying to get a few more minutes of shuteye, and the intrepid sailors left with abuse raining down on them from the upper floors.

Our boat was "The Merlin", a 30 ft trawler that looked decidedly unsafe and, as we lifted anchor to sail out of Durban harbour, someone almost fell overboard.

The sea was choppy with a scouring wind and before long Mike Grant was heaving over the side of the boat. Derek, arguably the most experienced sailor since he had travelled to the Antarctic, soon joined Mike in making disgusting gurgling sounds.

When we eventually dropped anchor, I expected everyone to look to me for instruction (since my tally as I pointed out earlier was in the hundreds of tons!), but I looked so youthful that the skipper, thinking that I was a child, had not brought a rod for me!

Sinkers had barely touched the seabed when everyone had to reel in and untangle their lines!

Soon serious fishing began. There was a loud shout from Derek as he struggled to reel in what turned out to be his heavy sinker.

Len Vermaak fought a raging battle with a large piece of seaweed, which the first mate helped him reel in.

Tony Hamilton landed a six-inch banana fish, but Derek, after recovering from another bout of seasickness, outdid him with an eight-inch Banana fish.

Eventually, the weather proved too much for us and, with all the lines heavily tangled, we called off the excursion.

Our total catch was 0.05 kg of fish – mostly inedible.

On our way back, one motor packed up, and the Merlin struggled back to port sounding like a buzz bike. A fuel pipe had burst and diesel fuel poured into the cabin, leading us to consider the need to radio for help.

However, we managed to limp home with the struggling motor, and the PYC[5] rescue team came to our assistance (but it was really unnecessary).

The experience was further marred when we reached the parking area: they had ticketed our cars for parking violations.

As promised, I must now explain how I became Durban's biggest fisherman.

---

[5] Point Yacht Club

Chapter 37

A Whale Of A Story

The radio operator on a whaling boat was a friend of my brother's and he invited me to join them on a trip. Whaling as an industry started in Durban in 1905 and was a thriving enterprise until 1975, but in 1982 the International Whaling Commission (IWC) established a moratorium on commercial whaling beginning in the 1985–86 season.

The eventual intention is to ban whaling in the southern oceans, which sounds pretty good to me.

I suppose most readers would agree with me that whaling is reprehensible, but please don't berate me for going on the trip.

I also apologise for the graphic details that follow – this story is certainly not for the squeamish. (If you have a weak stomach, perhaps you might prefer to skip this chapter or read it with your eyes closed.)

The boat belonged to the Union Whaling Company, and

I boarded it at the old whaling station near North Pier.

The captain was a tall, tanned Norwegian man with brilliant bright blue eyes and short blond hair. He spoke with a distinctive Scandinavian accent.

He showed me to my cabin below deck, which had a bunk and a fold-down metal table where I unpacked my things.

A few minutes later I joined the crew in the canteen.

We set sail at around 7pm and I watched the harbour lights disappear over the horizon. The starry sky without the smog and scatter of city lights looked spectacular, and I amused myself by identifying familiar constellations (such as the Southern Cross).

After a while I felt queasy and retired to my cabin, took a seasick tablet, which caused me to feel drowsy, and sank into watery oblivion.

Some hours later, I awoke to an eerie silence, except for the occasional lapping of water against the side of the boat. I peered out of the porthole and looked straight into the work sheds of Durban harbour.

We were back in port!

The captain had turned back because the weather had become inclement – and I had slept through it all.

The following evening, we set sail again, and it was then – no pun intended – plain sailing.

What a carefree life on board the whaler! When not performing their duties, crew members would recline on the deck, with others reading in the entertainment area on the deck below.

I had lengthy conversations with the captain, who removed his shirt to sport a long right paramedian laparotomy scar.

We were standing alongside the harpoon gun.

"What surgery was that?" I asked.

He smiled as he ran his calloused hand through his hair.

"It was done for what you doctors call a peptic ulcer," he grinned, showing yellowed teeth between his stubble.

At the time we associated peptic ulcers with stress, which seemed odd because he appeared perpetually relaxed.

Boy, was I wrong! When the sailor in the crow's nest spotted the spray from the blowhole of a monstrous mammal, all hell broke loose!

The captain manned the harpoon gun mounted at the bow, while gesticulating and yelling orders.

The uninitiated cannot grasp the drama of the chase that occurred after the man from aloft the crow's nest cried, "Blows!"

So, here's a blow-by-blow account of the first encounter.

The announcement over the intercom was ear-shattering.

"Sperm whale, sperm whale 200 metres."

The crew sprang into action, scattering in all directions, and the shirtless captain swung the harpoon gun around – essentially a canon with a large harpoon tied to a thick rope.

Through the cacophony, the radio continued, announcing various ASDIC (sonar) parameters: "Whale 10 degrees, 15 degrees, 20, 30…"and then "90 degrees 10 metres," which signified that the mammal was 10 metres directly under the boat.

It felt like ages before anything more happened (but was probably only about 15 minutes). Then the announcement came: "Whale 80 degrees, 70, 60, 50, 40" and then "5 degrees". This meant that the whale was surfacing.

Once the herd surfaced, they seemed content to swim alongside the boat – suggesting innocent trust.

Our captain, sporting various degrees of indecorous behaviour, swore obscenities with his orders. He looked for the largest of the herd – a cow – took aim with the gun and with a deafening bang a 165-pound harpoon flew through the air striking the whale.

The herd scattered, and the wounded whale tried to dive, but an extraordinary amount of thick rope attached to massive metal reels pulled at her, the ship's mast acting as a giant fishing rod and line.

As the whale's strength and energy waned, large motors reeled it in.

There was an ear-splitting explosion as the captain fired a grenade into the whale's head and the sea turned a bright red for metres around and the animal stopped thrashing.

The amount of blood was unimaginable and within minutes sharks appeared, circling the carcass and snapping off chunks of flesh. A sickening scene. (I warned you it would be graphic – sorry.)

The crew dragged the whale against the boat and plunged a long pipe with a sharpened end into it. They pumped compressed air into the lifeless torso, which then rose out of the water like a floating albatross. Then they drove another rod with a radio transmitter, red light and flag into the whale and cut the rope letting it drift away.

They killed 18 whales over the 3 days – each allowed to float away into the Indian Ocean.

On the last day and the trip home, we located the whales using the radio transmitter and receiver.

I ventured onto the deck one night to see the crew shackling a whale to the side of the boat. They were shining bright lights into the ocean, which attracted dozens – if not hundreds – of squid. These were hauled in as they clung to multicoloured tape and were later eaten by the crew.

We sailed into the harbour dragging 18 whale carcasses alongside to the whaling station on the seaward side of Durban's bluff.

It was a depressing yet mind-boggling experience.

Now you know why my tally was over 200 tons of fish.

I knew you wouldn't buy it unless I explained it.

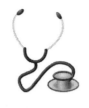

Chapter 38

Paediatric House Job and Starting GP

Addington Children's Hospital, a beautiful colonial-era building with a clock tower facing the Indian Ocean, was a great place to do my paediatric house job.

The amiable Dr Bill Winship was the chief of paeds. He had red-tinged hair and tortoiseshell broad-rimmed spectacles, and wore a perpetually knowing smile.

His department was exceedingly well run, and I got the impression that Christopher Good had put in a good word for me to get the senior houseman post in Winship's unit.

Looking after the little people, especially neonates, is challenging, and during my time there I developed a tremendous respect for the doctors who treat these tiny kids.

I was called one evening to see a six-month-old infant boy who was failing to thrive and had a distended abdomen. Over the previous two days, he had been anorexic but had been vomiting on and off from the age of two weeks.

He was mildly dehydrated with sunken eyes and a dry tongue, but it was the massive abdominal distention that caught my attention. I had the impression there was an intra-abdominal mass.

A common clinical diagnosis of such massive distention is Hirschsprung's disease, where colonic dilatation occurs because of a disturbance in the bowel neuroanatomy (so-called aganglionosis). Considering the size of the mass, I asked the registrar, Gerry Stiles, if a Wilm's tumour of the kidney was also a possibility.

I set up a drip and corrected his fluid and electrolyte levels, then ordered an X-ray of his abdomen. This caused my jaw to drop. *A vertebral column was clearly visible in the kiddie's abdomen!*

Those were the days before CT and I don't recall us using ultrasound.

The good-natured surgeon, Mr Jimmy Kirstein, examined the patient the next morning. We had a clear-cut case of a very rare disorder: foeto-in-foetus.

This little guy basically had his twin inside his abdomen, a parasitic twin foetus growing within its host – freakish!

An exploratory laparotomy was done and a large mass consisting of an anencephalic foetus, but also a separate teratoma, was removed. (This was considered by experts to be a third twin.)

A teratoma is a kind of growth that contains various tissue elements.

The case was recorded in the *SA Medical Journal* (vol 48, 1974) as the first case ever of foetus-in-foetus *and* teratoma.

Of course, foot soldiers don't feature in the accolades, so my name did not appear in the article, which saw Dr Winship, Mr Kirstein and the radiologist, Dr du Plessis, receiving a medal from the SA Medical Association.

Here is the abstract from the *SA Medical Journal.*

Fetus in fetu and Teratoma
JPG Du Plessis, WS Winship, JDL Kirkstein
Abstract

A case is reported in which a fetus in fetu and a malignant teratoma were present within the same intraabdominal mass in a 6-month-old male infant. It is the first record of such an occurrence, and attention is drawn to the possible significance of this case, in view of the now-rejected concept that a teratoma is the result of an abnormal process of twinning.

S. Afr. Med. J., 48, 2119 (1974)

During my stay in his department, Bill Winship made me realise why all medics should do a stint of paediatrics to acquire confidence in managing kids.

"Peter, are you interested in doing general practice?"

he once asked me.

Academic medicine fascinated me, but not general practice and I didn't want to be derailed from a career in clinical pharmacology. The paediatric job was a steppingstone to my planned return to Pretoria.

Despite this, Dr Winship was keen to introduce me to a GP with whom he had been in partnership before taking up paediatrics.

Drs G, G and A ran one of the largest and most successful general practices in Durban, with rooms in Salisbury Arcade in the city centre as well as in Montclair, about 20 km out of town.

Dr A had suffered from depression and had taken his life and the other Dr G had left for greener pastures. I wish I had contacted him before acting impetuously because it was no fun working there.

Dr Winship had said "glowing things" about me and insisted that I at least meet Dr G.

A week later I met the middle-aged and sullen Dr G, dressed in a light brown safari suit and shiny brown toe-capped shoes.

Winship introduced him to me and he allowed himself a brief smile before resuming the sullen stance. He feigned friendliness and espoused great things about his practice and the merits of family medicine. I remained uninterested but accepted a dinner invitation for the following Friday evening.

My girlfriend, Cheryl and I arrived in the yellow Alfa

GT and parked under the portico of Dr and Mrs G's opulent house in Anleno Road in the less affluent Montclair.

The chic furniture and expensive drapes impressed us, with the fine crystal glassware, beautiful, yet cold, reflecting the chandelier.

The aloof Mrs G tried hard to be hospitable and you could see that she wore the pants in the relationship.

She served us a three-course meal, and we dithered momentarily over a selection of wine. I stared intensely as the doctor tucked into his meal with gusto. There was clinking cutlery and awkward small talk. (Actually, hardly anyone chatted at the table apart from Dr G, who spoke with his mouth full.)

Pointing vaguely with his knife, he said: "You know, Peter, being a GP is just selling yourself to people."

I reached for my glass of claret, took a sip, and looked sideways at him, but I was appalled (faintly in the back of my mind, I thought about Dr Philip and his peashooter).

Dinner ended with an after-dessert sherry in the drawing room and I studied Dr G and the jut of his jaw as he drank.

He swirled the glass and drained his sherry. Then he got up and dropped a bombshell: "I will pay you one thousand rand a month until you become a full partner." He made a fist to emphasise the point.

I never saw that coming and almost spat out my sherry.

I gulped. It was like, "Oh my god!"

My salary as a medical officer was about R300 pm! But R1000... It was like catnip to a kitten!

Driving home, we discussed financial freedom (or how to get out of the Alfa Romeo debt trap).

A day later, Cheryl left a note for me: "So am I going to be a GP's wife or a pharmacologist's mistress?"

(When I had mentioned my plan to return to Pretoria, she had mentioned she might write to me.)[6]

While I should have thought it through, the following month I grasped the nettle, resigned my senior houseman post in paediatrics and joined Dr G.

I regretted the move.

---

[6] A few years later while practicing in Umhlanga Rocks, I managed to do the Masters in Clinical Pharmacology, but it meant I had to fly to Pretoria every Wednesday for three years. I genuinely think that they felt so sorry for me travelling the 500 km to Johannesburg and hiring a car from there to Pretoria, that they gave that qualification to me.
(A pity frequent flier rewards were unheard of at the time.)

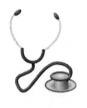

Chapter 39

Twin Delivery

It was a call no GP would relish.

I had just stepped out of the shower, wrapped only in a towel, when the phone rang.

Mother's Hospital needed me for a twin delivery and the charge sister was on the line.

Nowadays a GP would probably not deliver twins and a specialist obstetrician, knowing the complications, would opt for a caesarean section.

I managed a "What?"

Then, "Why are you calling me?"

"Dr G is away, and we see you are doing his calls."

The thought of delivering a patient that I had not cared for antenatally was daunting. A twin delivery scared me to death.

My mind raced. "Please give her 50 mg Pethidine and 25 mg Sparine," I said, my palms sweaty as I clutched the phone.

There was a prolonged silence, then she replied,

"Please repeat your order to my colleague."

I repeated the order, slammed down the phone and riffled through my medical books for my obstetric textbook – *Donald's Textbook of Obstetrics*.

I ran my finger down the alphabetic index to *Twin Delivery*.

Keep in mind that I had never done an obstetric house job (residency) – I went into general practice relying on my undergraduate training!

Luckily I had performed two twin vaginal deliveries and even a triplet delivery as a medical student at Kalafong Hospital – but that was under supervision.

The pages in Donald's textbook detailed the complications: more postpartum bleeds, cord prolapse, more abruptio, more uterine inertia and locked twins.

Yikes! Double the trouble.

I read it over and over, the sweat prickling my armpits.

I froze when the phone rang again and waited with my hand hovering over the receiver for the second ring, before lifting it.

It was the same sister from Mother's on the line.

"Hello, doctor, we need to talk."

"Sure, what's going on?" I bit my bottom lip.

"Doctor," she said, her tone authoritative and arrogant, "I don't care about your Pethidine and Sparine. You'd better just come."

I plonked down the phone, mustered Cheryl and, textbook in hand, rushed to the car.

While I drove, Cheryl read the steps of twin delivery aloud from the book!

I sprinted up the steps to the labour ward at Mother's Hospital in Greyville and greeted the nurse as I entered the room.

"I don't think I can do this," I whimpered.

She seemed to understand. "So why are you doing it?" she asked sympathetically.

"What else can I do?"

"Well, you could call a gynae [sic]."

I never knew it was that simple – merely call an obstetrician.

Reassured, my heart rate normalised.

The room was busy with trolleys and resuscitation equipment, and I greeted the woman, her large abdomen protruding from a white hospital gown.

I assessed her as a Para1 Grav 2 – about 38 weeks. Palpating her abdomen revealed that one twin was obviously a vertex, but I was uncertain about the other.

What if it was breech? Could I deliver it? I shuddered at the prospect of an intrapartum external version (where one attempts to turn the baby from the outside – something I had not done).

Dr G had expected a "normal" twin delivery.

Her membranes had ruptured while at home, and she was almost fully dilated.

Things were moving fast.

I stared at the wall clock. Her contractions were regular – two or three minutes apart. She yelled and her body shuddered with each contraction.

I slipped on sterile gloves and did a PV – I could feel that one twin was clearly a vertex presentation with the occiput thankfully anteriorly placed. It bothered me that I could feel what I assumed was the baby's finger alongside the head.

Was this kid trying to "Superman" himself out into the world?

Her BP was on the high side of normal but not a concern.

I set up an iv line and drew blood to "compat" for a blood transfusion if needed, then passed a catheter into the urethra and emptied some urine into a container.

There was no question of the luxury of an epidural, but she puffed happily at the Entanox, a mixture of oxygen and nitrous oxide ($N2O$), which a patient could self-deliver with a mask. The $N2O$ is a valuable analgesic, and the oxygen reduces the risk of hypoxia.

As I write this, I recall sitting in the duty room at Mother's a few months later. I was waiting for a woman in labour to dilate and noticed the cylinder of Entanox. There was no one around so I tried a few puffs of the gas.

After a few deep breaths, my head began to swim, and the next thing I knew someone was shaking my shoulders and calling my name.

I opened my eyes to see the sister bending over me and prodding, "Doctor, doctor, are you okay?"

Cut back to my story...

We had phoned Dr Peter Perrot, and I was relieved to see him arrive. I called out to him, "Boy, am I glad to have you here. We need an expert and there's no one better!"

Waving away the compliment, he extended a hand.

"What's the problem?" Peter Perrot sounded reassuring.

I could only blurt out, "I'm not thrilled about this."

He put his hand on my lower back and led me to the patient, saying, "Relax, my boy."

He was my lifesaver.

"She's 90% effaced, just a rim of cervix and both vertex," he said, after examining the woman.

His eyes beaming, he added: "I'll pull up a chair against the wall and watch you do the delivery. I'll help when you need me. Tell me, what's the first thing you're going to do?"

"Check the babies' heartbeats – if I can."

"Then?"

"Time the contractions?"

He grabbed the chair, "I like it. Keep going."

The woman's guttural grunt announced the onset of each contraction and, sensing it was time to push, with her legs up in stirrups, I urged her on.

Her face went red and her neck veins protruded as she strained, and suddenly a head was crowning.

I injected local anaesthetic along the stretched area of her perineal flesh and called out to her to stop pushing.

Then I reached for the episiotomy scissors and cut at an angle along the stretched tissue.

Suddenly the head appeared, the face blue and pointing to the ground, and the baby slid into my hands.

It was a boy! I clamped and cut the cord and handed the baby to the efficient and experienced midwife.

There was a reassuring cry and his face glowed pink.

Peter Perrot was alongside me as we delivered the placenta and prepared for the second twin.

Auscultating with the old-fashioned Pinhard foetal stethoscope, which is essentially a metal horn, I picked up the reassuring foetal heartbeat. (No electronic or internal foetal and foetal heart monitoring in those days – heck, not even hand-held Doppler.)

The time between twins is critical but, lady luck being on my side, within five minutes the mother pushed again. I felt for the membrane and ruptured it with a Kocher's forceps. There was an impressive gush of fluid and the second twin emerged – also face-down.

Two boys – one just over 4 lbs and the other just over 5 lbs.

Remembering my grilling by Prof. Frans Geldenhuys about the dangers of a postpartum haemorrhage, I think I was lucky because PPH is a real issue in multiple births.

And thank goodness I did not need to attack the father with those Wrigley forceps.

(Of course, my bill could cause paternal poverty – one of the P's mentioned below.)

The chapter on complications of "multiple delivery" highlighted the many complications, which, interestingly, all begin with the letter P.

(You might need that medical dictionary again.)

More Pyelitis in pregnancy, more Pre-eclampsia, more Phlebitis, more Pernicious vomiting, more Placenta Praevia, more Placental abruption, more Postpartum bleeding, more Prolapsed cord, more Perineum laceration, more Perambulatory problems and, of course, the Paternal poverty I referred to.

I wanted to add: more Problems for Peter (not Perrot – me!).

The lesson learnt is: when your back is to the wall, get help. (Get Peter – but not any Tom, Dick or Harry.)

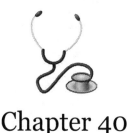

Chapter 40

The Aeronautical Engineer – Fun Leaks

Mr P, a retired aeronautical engineer, had a urological procedure that left him dribbling urine. He had initially presented with an inability to pee because of his large prostate gland.

The prostate gland sits below the bladder and the urethra (the tube that takes urine from the bladder), passes through the middle of the gland.

It always amazed me that nature designed things this way. Either evolution was wacky or the creator had a mean streak.

If there's one thing in the human body that's really been badly designed, it's the plumbing. You are guaranteed to develop voiding problems in your old age. (But then again, even women, who don't have the same pesky gland, also get problems.)

There is an old joke about God being a civil engineer,

because "who else would run a sewerage system through a recreational area?"

Mr P was freaked out by his urologist's suggestion that he use a sanitary towel.

"I'm a goddamn engineer!" he blurted out. "How can I use a woman's pad?"

Puzzled by the engineer part of his reasoning, I pointed out that it was only temporary.

He phoned the practice a few days later, insisting that he see me because he wanted to show me "something interesting".

As he entered my office, I spotted a wet stain on his pants. Without batting an eyelid, he lifted one leg of his trousers a few inches and removed a cork from a pipe jutting out from his pants. Some urine splashed onto the floor causing me to jump clear as it splattered my ankles.

"What the...!" I exclaimed, moving further away.

He unbuttoned his trousers and dropped them to the ground so that they bunched around his ankles.

Around his waist was an old-fashioned ladies' suspender belt. This was attached to the top part of a plastic bleach bottle cut through and inverted to serve as a funnel, with his penis dangling into the funnel. A black washing machine outlet pipe was attached to the bottle and extended all the way down his leg, with a cork blocking the end.

So, this was better than submitting to the indignity of

a simple sanitary pad!

The apparatus looked absurd, but, showing some enthusiasm, I remarked that it looked interesting.

"Quite nifty," I said.

His frown gave way to a wide-ranging smile. "Could you get the urologist to see my invention?" he asked.

In those days I was in awe of a specialist, and I suggested that he let me show a photograph to the urologist for his comment.

He phoned a week later inquiring about the specialist's opinion and if he could "mass produce" his device for the marketplace.

The photo had not yet been developed, so I sidestepped the issue and told him that the urologist's response had been tepid, and he had dismissed it as being unwieldy.

There was a long silence and after checking that he was still on the line I added, "Perhaps you could improve the design."

Obviously miffed at having his invention spurned, he put down the phone with a humph.

Later that week, my wife collected the camera for my son's second birthday party and handed the roll of film to a local pharmacy to be developed and prints made.

A week later (yes, that's how long we waited for our photos in the early seventies) she called to collect the pictures only to be told by the pharmacist, Robbie Wright, that he could not print them because the developed film contained pornography!

"It can't be my film," the wife blurted.

"Oh yes it is," retorted Robbie. Then, adding a mischievous streak, he said, "Look at the images of your kids on the same strip of film!"

I got a phone call during a busy consulting morning to "please explain!".

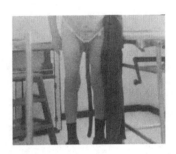

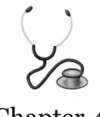

Chapter 41

"Who pulls the plug?"
And "Always bathe with
a friend"

I had just finished supper when the phone rang.

"Hello," I said, picking up the receiver.

"Hello, is that the doctor?" the voice was calm and composed.

"Yes, can I help?"

"Is that you, doctor?"

"Yes," I replied again, a bit irritated.

"Well, doctor, my name is Smith, and I wonder if you could help me?"

"Yes, what's the trouble...?"

"Well, doctor, it's my wife...," his voice trailed away.

"Yes, what's her problem?"

"Doctor, I think... I think she could be dead."

Jolted, I croaked, "Quick, give me your address."

Now call me crazy, but if someone *thinks* his wife is dead, then perhaps, just maybe, she could still be alive.

I called Cheryl to join me (as a trained nurse she could help with resuscitation) and raced to 73 Roland Chapman Drive, Montclair.

I sped up the road,71, 75, 77... I reversed and went up again 71,75, 77 but no 73!

A tall, tanned man was standing on the sidewalk, staring into space.

Cheryl opened her window, and I leant over and called to him.

"Excuse me, where is number 73?"

He held up a cigarette. "Sorry, but I'm not from this area."

I asked him to move over a few inches, and there behind him was the number 73. It was a panhandle driveway! (A panhandle is a property squeezed between two properties, with the house placed well back at the end of a long narrow driveway.)

I raced up the driveway and when I cut the engine, it continued to turnover (so-called "pre-ignition"), delaying my exit from the car.

Stepping over a runnel of water, I dashed towards the house and I yelled back at Cheryl, "Stay in the car until I need you."

A few people sat silently on chairs and also on a low front wall of the veranda.

As I stepped onto the porch, a tall man stood up and stared down at me.

His poker face was so expressionless, he might as well have been in a coma for all the life it showed.

"Are you the doctor?" His voice was hoarse, and his breath smelt of smoke.

"Uh uh," I responded.

Then seemingly unperturbed and talking slowly, he waved an arm to the crowd: "This is my friend John, my brother Jake and his wife Mary."

"Hello, hello, hello," I blurted out in staccato speech. Then added, "Where is your wife?"

He turned towards the front door and took long languid strides down the passage toward the bathroom.

With my black medical bag at my side, I trailed behind him, attempting to keep up with the lengthy strides.

He pushed open the bathroom door.

Lying in the bath was a middle-aged lady, submerged and obviously dead. She was naked, her wide-open eyes staring up at the ceiling.

It did not escape my notice that nobody had thought to remove the plug. The water level was near the rim of the bathtub. The water was cold.

"She's dead," I mumbled.

He leant in and seemed not to understand what I had said.

"I said, 'she's dead'," I repeated.

"I thought she could be."

I suppose it was not professional, but I screamed at him. "You *thought* she's dead...? You never even let the water out!"

A few minutes passed then he asked, "What do we do now?" His voice was gravelly.

The TV series, Columbo, with Peter Falk as the eccentric detective with his rumpled brown overcoat and his signature line: *"There's just one more thing"*, was current at the time.

I straightened my white safari jacket and pulled the collar over my ear, looking as if I had just walked off the set of Columbo.

He must have been alarmed when I responded, "Call the police!"

So, I called the police.

Two uniformed officers arrived, a black man and a shorter middle-aged white guy, and I directed them to the bathroom, where they studied the scene.

"Can you pull the plug and get her out of the bath?" asked the shorter guy.

"Hey, I'm five foot two, nowhere near as big as you," I objected. "You get her out."

The unfortunate woman had suffered from epilepsy and had convulsed in her morning bath while the family were out for the day.

The maid had arrived at 9am and knocked repeatedly on the door. When there was no response, she'd left.

Their kids came home from school at 3.30pm and, finding themselves locked out, went to play at the neighbours.

It was only when the husband arrived at 6pm and managed to unlock the door that he found the wife in the bath.

If you'll stay with me on this, there is a message we can add: *It is a cruel irony that the doctor is always the one who is called upon to pull the plug in a hopeless case, bringing the reality of medicine into sharp focus.*

And, oh, just one more thing – when you are frail, don't bathe alone.

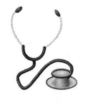

Chapter 42

Flattering Calls and The Drunk

The phone rang.

At the other end was a very inebriated man.

"Hello doctor," he slurred. "Can, can you help me, I sh... Sh...really need help. I...it's this Whiiiisssssky..."

"Yes, it does sound like you need help. What's the problem?"

He burped a few times then stumbled on, "I juz need lots of help, help, 'ow about you... I've vomited... Come see it?"

Captivated, I enquired, "Well, where are you?"

"I'm, I on corner of...of...er Prince an Mark street."

"Yes, but where is that?"

"South beach! corner Prrrinsan Marc."

"But where are you?"

"Izee you lika whi...whi...whissky too... I...on

corner..."

"But is it a house, a flat or a hotel?" I tried to conceal my irritation.

He mumbled: "It's a call box!"

A week before a lady had called me.

"Hello Dr Desmarais," she said. "It's so good to chat with you. I've heard some wonderful things about you."

"Well, that's kind of you, but I'm just doing my job."

"No, really, you have an amazing reputation..."

"Thanks, but..."

"No, I mean it. Everyone says..."

I felt encouraged as my head swelled but my ego quickly diminished when she completed her sentence:

"Everyone says that you are so good..."

She paused then added the clanger,

"...at dealing with drunks!"

How flattering.

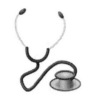

Chapter 43

I'LL GET HIM

It happened again, another one of those evening calls. This time I had just drifted off when the phone rang. On the line I could hear the frantic pleas of a woman – another damsel in distress.

"Doctor, help, oh please help me...!"

"Who is it...what's wrong?" My hand gripped the receiver.

The voice was breathless and panicky: "Help me! It's my bloody husband. The bastard's trying to kill me!"

Her voice pitched into a frenzied crescendo, "My name is Mrs R from number xx Clarence Rd. Someone help! Quickly."

The echoes of her screaming still ringing in my ears, I wanted to tell the damsel that, at five foot two, I was an unlikely knight, and she should phone the police, but she had already dropped the receiver.

I phoned "Squad cars" – the emergency police rescue service popularised at the time by a radio programme every Friday night on Springbok radio. Each episode would begin with a dramatic voice sound bite: "They prowl the empty streets at night..."

The cop offered to meet me at the patient's house and, with the excited Cheryl in tow, I raced off to the given address.

I had just parked the Alfa when the squad car – its light flashing – swerved in alongside me and I greeted the two officers as we entered the house.

The passage was strewn with newspapers and stubbed out cigarettes and, behind a closed door, a gut-wrenching noise echoed through the building. A woman was shouting.

We bashed open the door and entered a small and cluttered room that smelt of stale and damp air. Here we encountered a thin unshaven middle-aged man in shorts and vest wielding a broken bottle.

A woman in her late 40s was cowering under a cup-board shelf, with the hostile man brandishing the jagged end of the bottle at her face. She kept shooting her leg out, while trying to cover her face with an arm. The man, who smelt of booze, had her other arm tightly wedged against the cupboard.

The cop grabbed the assailant at the back of his neck and pulled him forwards. As he lost his balance, the officer overpowered him and wrestled the bottle from his grip, allowing the distraught woman to break away from him like a freed animal.

She flopped to the ground, her eyes red and her face

mascara-stained.

It was gut wrenching.

The man with the woman now out of his clutches, swung at me and I dodged backwards just missing his fist, but the officer grabbed his arm and handcuffed it behind him.

Steering him out to the driveway, the cop prompted him to get into the car.

The prisoner then turned and, noticing the wife sitting in the Alfa Romeo, signalled that he wanted to "talk to the doctor's wife".

At first the officer refused, then relented, and, with the cuffed man tightly in his clutches, he led him to the Alfa.

Cheryl lowered her window a few inches, and the guy pushed his face menacingly against the window and sneered, "Are you the slime ball doctor's wife?"

She recoiled from his booze breath, bit her bottom lip and nodded.

"I'll get your bastard husband!" he snorted through clenched teeth.

Cheryl quickly locked the door.

I ran up to the man and floored him in a rugby tackle, twisted his right arm behind him and bashed his head against the ground.

Okay, I didn't really do that, but you can imagine that I wished I could.

They bundled Mr R into the squad car and took him to the local police station, where it became apparent that we had picked the wrong establishment to take him to.

With two constables, I accompanied him to Entabeni Hospital and admitted him to a medical ward, prescribed a strong sedative and planned to get a psychiatrist to see him in the morning.

They assigned a constable to keep watch over Mr R.

I was in the front office, completing the admission documents, when a nurse came crying that Mr R had escaped custody.

So we organised a search with nursing staff and the police, looking through the wards and the front parking lot.

I had a torch in hand and scurried about the bushes facing the parking lot looking for the guy.

But while I was waving my flashlight back and forth, amongst the trees, it occurred to me that *"this was the man who wanted to get me!"*

So much for taking him away in a straitjacket. But not being a total moron, I knew it was time to hit my bed, and I went home.

There was a call from the police the following morning. The psychotic Mr R had been apprehended and committed to the psychiatric hospital in Pictermaritzburg.

I heard nothing further about the contentious Mr R.

A few months passed, and one Saturday morning we picnicked in the salty air on the lawn alongside the slipway at the Bluff Yacht Club.

My mother-in-law, Marge, and my siblings-in-law were enjoying the day, lounging on a blanket with snacks, cans of lager and cool drinks, when a small Jack Russell dog meandered over, sniffing our food.

A Volkswagen Kombi from the 1960s was parked alongside us. The owner, a thin man in his early fifties, heavily tattooed and with his sleeves rolled high on his arms, was relaxing in a camping chair in front of his wagon.

Each time the dog wandered onto our blanket, he would scuttle across, lift the dog and apologise for the intrusion.

We weren't really disturbed and assured him that we were animal lovers.

He was courteous, but there was something about the guy – you know, that feeling.

He had been eyeing Marge for most of the afternoon and, after a while, sauntered over to ask if she would go with him on his yacht.

Marge politely declined the offer, but the man was insistent.

We urged her to go, saying, "Come on, he seems a nice guy – you'll enjoy a cruise around the harbour."

She eased her lips into a smile, seemed embarrassed, but then relented and let him lead her to the slipway.

As they donned their lifejackets and Marge embarked, I could feel my search engine overheating.

Where? Where? – scouring the recesses.

He led her onto his craft and the wind swept them

away into the turquoise ocean extending in all directions to the horizon.

The sun was dripping down with the sail silhouetted against a remarkable sunset and I still could not stop myself thinking about where I had met the guy.

As they sailed off, it hit me – Mr R! – from the Squad car drama!

Oops. Was I in hot water? Wow – encouraging my mother-in-law to go to sea with this madman. (What right-thinking person would do this?)

Luckily, Mom enjoyed her trip and returned safely and Mr R no longer bore any resentment.

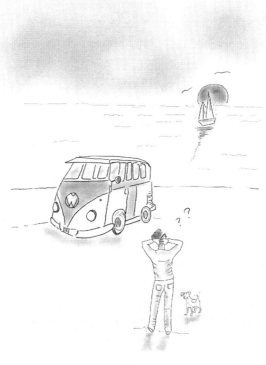

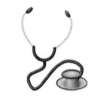

Chapter 44

The Fickle Finger of Fate

In February 1974, I joined the Venniker, Pickford and Partners practice with offices in Field Street, Durban and also Bartle Road in the Umbilo area.

We took turns consulting on Sundays at the Bartle Road rooms. It was Tony Venniker's turn, but, since something unforeseen had popped up, he asked me to do his call.

Tony was hugely popular, but it annoyed me to see that he had 100 patients booked on that day!

(It was enough to make a batsman smile – a century on Sunday!)

Tony had an uncanny belief in vitamin injections, and many patients came just for a B12 shot. Some came for other injectable medications (shot-happy patients who become dependent and devoted to shot-happy doctors).

You would've thought that only the really sick people would arrive on Sunday, but many wanted BP checks and repeat prescriptions.

(Many quick singles.)

Once again, one risks not caring, just to clear the crowds.

It's this issue of not caring that can hit you like an invisible bus after years of hard work. Some doctors see their role as recognising pathology and referring on – see and turf – not exactly what I had aspired to when I chose to do medicine.

I sat at my desk and was asking myself how I had got caught up in this predicament, when a large middle-aged woman in a simple floral dress plopped herself down in front of me.

"I've come for a medical check-up," she said.

I resented the imposition. How unreasonable – on a Sunday – for a check-up.

I locked eyes with her.

"But it's Sunday," I berated her, "What do you want checked?"

"Just a little check-up," she replied.

"Do you have any symptoms – complaints?"

"Not really."

"Well, should I check your heart?"

"Yes."

"What about your lungs?"

"Yes."

"And your liver, stomach, kidneys, ears, eyes, spine? How about testing for diabetes or how your thyroid is functioning...?"

By then it should've dawned on her that there was really no such thing as *a little check-up.*

I decided to humour her. I took a brief history and told her to remove her dress, but not her undergarment.

A cursory general examination, including listening to her heart and lungs, was normal.

"Lie on your side and pull down your drawers."

Her face flushed.

"What for?" she stammered.

I slipped on a glove. "I need to put my finger up your bum."

"Is that really necessary?" She was indignant and wrinkled up her nose in defensive disgust.

My reply was smug. "Well, that's part of a check-up," I said. "They teach you at medical school that if you don't put your finger in it, you put your foot in it!"

(I needed to teach her a lesson for coming on Sunday.)

She shut her eyes tight, turned on her side, and flexed her butt cheeks.

I slipped my gloved finger in and the tip struck a firm mass.

"Have you had any change in bowel habit?" I asked, slipping off the gloves with two snapping sounds.

She had a tear in her eye when she conceded that she did indeed experience discomfort after defecation.

I arranged for a surgeon to see her the following day, for what turned out to be an operable (so curable) cancer of the rectum.

A little check-up; seriously, what does it even mean?

But sticking to a little check-up might result in a little bit of death.

So that is the art of medicine.

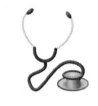

Chapter 45

You Can't Trust Your Memory

I took off a Friday to sort out a tax issue at the Receiver of Revenue offices at the bottom of Smith Street.

The useless public servant who served me couldn't help me and to my chagrin wanted me to return on another day with further documentation.

As I left the building, I almost collided with an elderly man shuffling along the sidewalk.

I didn't recognise him at first, but then he pulled down his sunglasses.

"Mr Edwards!" I exclaimed, and since I thought I knew him and recalled his name I could not resist exchanging pleasantries.

(This has seldom happened to me and it felt good having something to say.)

"How are you?" I asked.

"Yes, yes. I'm very well, doctor," he answered.

There was silence and I felt uneasy.

"You look well. You've made a good recovery," I said and steered him over to a quiet corner.

His eyes narrowed. "No, no, I wasn't ill. It was my wife! You looked after her..."

" Oh yes," I responded, "Of course, how could I forget! How is she now?"

"No, you were there when she died!" he shot back.

"You held her hand when she took her last breath."

At that moment, I wished that the pavement would swallow me up.

He reminded me again that I was in the bedroom with her when she passed away.

I vowed never ever to assume anything when seeing a patient out of context.

But the lesson is never learnt – perhaps it's my lack of memory for names and faces, or possibly just because as a doctor one encounters many people in a short time.

It makes me want to wear a hoodie going to a shopping mall.

(A Darth Vader cape and Samurai helmet might suit me fine.)

I was at the airport with my wife waiting to meet a friend arriving from Johannesburg.

A large crowd had gathered in the waiting area and, in the distance, an old lady waved at me.

I waved back and, not recognising the woman, I beckoned to the wife to move across so that I did not need to confront the woman. But the crowds had crammed us in, and I could see the old lady trying desperately to get closer.

I tried to push further back and, with the crowds swaying and shifting, I urged my wife to move along with me. I really didn't feel like chatting to the lady.

Then the wife blurted, "Where's this old lady?"

"There," I said, pointing to her. "Let's move before she gets closer, I haven't a clue who she is."

My wife craned her neck to look over the crowds and then announced, "That's my granny!"

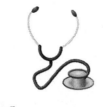

Chapter 46

Gunshot after Midnight

It was pouring, and I awoke to the phone ringing between the thunder and the flashes of lightning illuminating the bedroom. I held the receiver to my ear. It was past midnight, and the distraught lady caller announced that she had just shot herself.

I sat bolt upright in bed.

"What happened?" I asked as I wiped the sleep from my eyes.

Someone had told her that when the weather was inclement, bullets in a gun could explode. While she'd been removing the bullets from the magazine in the storm, the pistol had discharged into her lower abdomen. She was in no pain and felt okay.

I flicked on the light, looked for my trousers and riffled through my bedside drawer for my keys, then hastily dressed and within minutes was steering my blue Volvo 164 to a flat in Bartle Road. (The yellow Alfa sports had given way to the bigger sedan – better to accommodate a wife and a child – so more debt.)

I parked in the street and stepped onto the wet pavement. Across the street the individual flats were in darkness and the hazy streetlamps cast long shadows. I gripped my little black bag tightly as I bounded up the steps.

The front door was ajar, with a hallway light flickering across the stairwell.

As I entered, I was surprised to see her sitting comfortably on an upright kitchen chair in the centre of her living room.

Her right arm was draped across her body, clasping the opposite elbow, with a small calibre pistol resting on her lap. She appeared calm.

With her vital signs appearing normal, I patted down her torso and legs, looking for an injury and blood.

There was a fingernail-sized entrance wound just above her pubic area, with a small stream of blood trickling downwards.

She needed hospital admission and, grateful for the roomier car, I took her to St Augustine's in the Volvo. (With arms outstretched, the statue of Jesus near the reception area now seemed to welcome us.)

Once admitted we set up an iv line, and did the required blood studies and compat, in case she needed blood.

On both the straight abdominal and the lateral X-ray, one could see the bullet in the middle of the pelvis. There was no free air.

So the bullet was "slap bang" in the middle of the pelvis.

There was a trace of blood in her urine at dipstick test, indicating bladder injury or even other internal organ damage, so it was clear that she needed surgical exploration and I phoned Roy Wise.

It was almost 2am, and the kindly sister suggested I take a nap on one of the side-room beds while waiting for Roy.

I closed my eyes and drifted off.

I had just nodded off when someone tugging at my toe shook me awake. "Mr Wise is here to see your patient," said a junior nurse.

Roy was sipping tea in the duty room. "Hello Peter, why don't you examine your patients properly?" he chided.

He held out his hand to display a dull grey metal object.

The bullet!

I rubbed my eyes with my fists and yawned. Narrowing my eyes, I checked my watch. Had I slept through the operation?

It was 2.15am. They said Roy was fast, but he couldn't have done the surgery in ten minutes!

He blew on his tea then grinned.

"I did a vaginal examination, as all surgeons worth their mettle should, and there was the bullet!"

How weird – imagine that, removing the bullet from the vagina!

So, it's not only a finger in your bum that can save your life.

At the obligatory laparotomy, we closed holes in the bladder, small bowel and vaginal fornix.

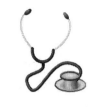

Chapter 47

Part-time Surgery

Urban private practice can be uninteresting because of the scarcity of interesting pathology, so craving diversion I had a thought.

I took the lift to Dr Good's office on the 12th floor at Addington Hospital to ask about a part-time post in the department of internal medicine and, as we stopped on the first floor, Alan White, chief of surgery, stepped in.

As I mentioned earlier, he used to call me Petrushka.

"So where are you going, Petrushka?" he asked now.

"Hi Mr White, I'm off to see Dr Good for a part-time job in medicine," I answered.

"Nonsense," he said. "You're coming to my office for a surgical post."

It was more a threat than a statement.

"No, no," I remonstrated, "I would rather work in medicine."

Shoving his forefinger against my lips, he steered me out of the lift and into his office on the third floor.

He sat behind his desk, his lean and tall frame outlined by the sunlight streaming through the window. Rummaging through some papers, he thrust an application-for-a-post form in front of me. He lifted the phone and mumbled something incomprehensible to the staff office but carried on talking to me with the phone against his ear.

He wouldn't take "no" for an answer and shook the phone at me, saying, "Sign here."

Within minutes I was signing an application as a part-time medical officer in the department of surgery.

It was a bugger being on surgical call one night a week at Addington and certainly no fun when your only training was a six-month surgical house job.

If you ran into trouble such as encountering some other intra-abdominal catastrophe while doing a simple appendicectomy, you'd better know what to do.

One evening, a patient in his mid-fifties presented with an abdominal wound.

During an altercation, his jilted lover had stabbed him with a large kitchen knife. (I probably missed Haranimus's lecture about how important it was to know the size of the knife as this could give one an idea of the extent of the injury.)

The patient was stable and seemed comfortable but had a loop of intestine hanging out in front of his belly.

The casualty officer had set up an IV line, done the

usual blood work and ordered compatibility testing in case the patient required a blood transfusion.

It was my call that evening, and I studied the X-ray, which showed air trapped under the diaphragm – the tell-tale sign of a hollow organ injury. (This is commonly referred to as "free air," meaning air in the belly outside of the confines of the intestine.)

I didn't think I could do the case and phoned Mr Alan White.

"Yes, Petrushka. What's the problem?" he asked.

"This guy has bowel evisceration and I don't think I can do it alone," I said.

I could almost feel him shaking his head.

"Nonsense, my boy, do a right paramedian incision and close any holes with a 441 suture."

"But..."

His voice was too determined for any rebuttal.

He had already put the phone down.

I drew in a deep breath.

At the operating table, the houseman looked relaxed, oblivious to my anxiety.

I made a large incision down the centre of the abdomen from the sternum down around the umbilicus.

It's a satisfying feeling slicing through skin and fat, and a simple matter to open the parietal peritoneum and peer into the abdominal cavity.

Fifteen years earlier, I had done this on frogs in my bedroom laboratory without having any idea of what I was looking at.

I lifted a loop of small bowel and found a gaping hole through the layers of intestine. I remembered the 441 instruction, and the forceps, loaded with the suture, got slapped into my hand.

I closed the hole and lifted more bowel – there were two more holes!

While preoccupied with the holes, I didn't notice a second iv line running blood with the anaesthetist squeezing bags of blood into the patient. His BP had dropped precipitously, and the anaesthetist was yelling instructions to his floor staff and then at me.

"What about his spleen?"

At the anaesthetist's suggestion, I ran my hand over the spleen – it felt smooth and healthy.

Then I felt the part of the liver I could reach and it too seemed okay.

I was sweating, but steadied my nerves by talking.

I asked for the special plastic bag that is used to isolate the intestines (bowel bag).

The bowel floats free within the peritoneum like a bunch of snakes in a bag. (Think of the peritoneum as the bag holding these snakes.)

But it is still attached to the back wall of the abdomen by its mesentery so you can empty the intestines into the bowel bag while they remain attached to the body.

To my horror the posterior peritoneum was bulging!

The thought crossed my mind: *Oh, my god, the bloody knife probably passed through the aorta causing a massive posterior peritoneal bleed!* (The aorta sits behind the peritoneum, which envelopes the intestines.)

I shoved the bowel back into the abdominal cavity, held a large wet swab against the organs and, going white, (excuse the pun) yelled: "Get Mr White!"

Alan White lived in Durban North. He was scrubbed and beside me within 15 minutes – how the heck he did this I will never know.

"Now, now, my boy," he said, "Don't panic."

I muttered, "This is big boy surgery." But cool as a cucumber, he opened the posterior peritoneum.

He divided the layers to expose the retroperitoneal structures, while I suctioned blood and clots.

The knife had passed through the upper pole of the left kidney, severed the superior mesenteric artery and landed in the substance of the pancreas.

We tied off bleeders and sutured the kidney, and suddenly the BP came up from close to zero.

Alan White made surgery look like darning your socks.

It was indeed big boy surgery, and my boots were much too small!

(And my bladder had learnt to contain itself for eight hours.)

Later in the change room Alan White smiled, "It's more fun when there's drama."

We finished at 4am and I got home at 5.30am just as my wife was waking up.

I had misjudged and couldn't handle the case, and Cheryl said I should resign.

General practice and part-time surgery just don't mix.

I'm not sure why I delayed writing my letter of resignation. I just procrastinated. The days became weeks, and the weeks months, and I continued with the surgical call.

Some months later, an official envelope marked "Addington Hospital, Dept of Surgery" landed on my desk.

It could only mean one thing: a call to abandon my post (in effect firing me) because of surgical ineptitude, so the envelope remained unopened until sunset when I tore it open.

My jaw dropped. It wasn't what I was expecting (neither was it business class tickets to the Grand Prix in Monaco though).

"Dear Dr Desmarais, it is with pleasure that I inform you that we have allocated you the post of senior surgeon with the following remuneration..."

A senior surgeon had resigned, and Alan White had recommended that they give the post with its better pay to me.

I waited three months and then resigned, but kept the letter – it made for an impressive CV.

There's a certain allure about being able to do surgery

– you can always go and swing a golf club, but Tiger Woods can never operate.

Another cheat...

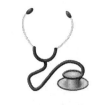

Chapter 48

Shark Attack

People are funny. They hate standing in queues. On reaching the front of the queue, though, some sort of strange metamorphosis occurs. They suddenly have all day and the impatient queue behind them falls off into another dimension. Empathy deficiency is rife.

Here's a thing: have you ever considered that sometimes your doctor might struggle to wrap up a consultation? I mean, it's not as easy as saying: "Your time's up!"

Occasionally I'd get stuck with a loquacious retiree, his arm over the back of the chair, discussing world affairs or the stock market. As he rambled on, I would fidget impatiently with my stethoscope bell, clicking it from side to side.

I could sit it out and not comment, hoping that once he realised he was encroaching on another's time, he would leave.

After some time of enduring this, I had an idea. Over

a weekend, I installed a buzzer in the reception area linked to a hidden button under my desk that could alert the front office to my plight!

An astute receptionist could then feign a "minor emergency".

I'd inherited my receptionist, Robin from Derek van Deventer. She was a short plump woman, religious and as honest as the day is long – someone who could never tell a lie.

Cocking her head, she stared incredulously at my installation.

Her eyes followed the cable leading under the carpet from a button under my desk along the passage to the reception area, where it connected to a buzzer.

If I lifted my knee, it would buzz.

"What must I do when it rings?" She gave me a questioning look like we were in cahoots to eavesdrop on the President.

"You need to make a scene with some excuse for the patient to leave."

"But I'd have to lie!"

"Robin, it's for a good cause – it will help the practice run on time."

You would have thought it was the equivalent of invading Iraq.

The look that crept across her face was akin to what you would see on a nun's face after you had suggested she might wear a bikini to the next Eucharist and, perhaps, if the spirit moved her, twerk a little.

Some months later after completing a consultation, a patient decided it was time to chat about the economy.

He rambled on and on and on and on.

This was my chance – I raised my knee and bumped the buzzer while he was expounding on interest rates and inflation.

There was a distant buzz.

Robin barged in, facing me and stood behind the seated patient.

She was panting, cheeks red and the veins in her neck popping out.

"Doctor...doctor", she squeezed out.

I wanted to laugh but, trying to look serious, I said, "Yes, Robin, what is it?"

It is common knowledge that not everyone can wink. Robin had never learnt to do this without drawing up the corner of her mouth in a sort of grimace.

"Doctor, doctor," her face contorting, she said, "It's a... It's a...shark attack!"

I choked...

My rooms were 100 metres from the Umhlanga beach, and her choice of a suitable minor emergency was a shark attack!

"Shark attack," my voice was falsetto. "Robin, are you sure?"

Robin was hyperventilating, her face doing the fandango.

"Yes, yes – the teeth – at the beach. A shark has attacked someone!"

Annoyed, I leapt up.

"I must go!"

The patient jumped up, "Shit, a shark attack, I'm with you!"

My mind raced. "No, no, you stay here!" I instructed him. "Let me check what's going on."

I turned away to hide my embarrassment and left, slamming the door behind me.

As soon as we were out of earshot, I pulled Robin aside.

"Why a shark attack? Don't you realise I have to leave these rooms and go to the damn beach? And everyone will want to read about it in the papers!" I almost yelled.

She sobbed, "Sorry, sorry."

I thought quickly. Just outside my office, but within earshot of my patient, was a phone.

I lifted the silent handpiece. "Oh, okay," I feigned, "glad to hear that."

And I hung up after a "Uh, huh."

My patient was shuffling impatiently in his chair and did the "My god, what's happening?" thing as I returned to the office.

"It's a false alarm," I tried to look confident, "Someone's been injured on the beach, but Dr van Deventer is there helping, so I'm not needed."

He tipped his head back and roared with laughter, then he slumped backward and made himself comfortable.

A slick smile spread across his face, "Well, you certainly have a fascinating life! It reminds me of when..."

And, dear reader, I had to sit through another story.

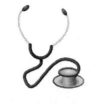

Chapter 49

Vitamins Or Pet Food

Mrs Dale had essential hypertension and saw me every six months for an assessment of her blood pressure control.

On one occasion, she asked me to suggest a good vitamin preparation to use as a regular supplement.

I doubt very much if the average person on a healthy diet requires vitamin supplementation – something we could debate at some length.

Vitamins are obviously necessary dietary constituents needed in tiny quantities to act as regulators or catalysts in biochemical reactions.

But they are no more necessary than carbohydrates, fats, proteins, electrolytes and minerals, and let's face it, they don't have the magical properties that people want to attribute to them.

Yes, they are ESSENTIAL. But so are all nutrients.

Remove sodium from your diet and you will die. The

same goes for calcium, magnesium, cobalt, iron and hundreds of other substances.

The problem, I think, relates to the lofty name, Vitamin, given to this group of chemicals. This happened because the first substances discovered were amines that were considered essential for life; they enjoyed the label **Vital Amines** or vitamines. (Later when they established that there were other substances that were not amines, they dropped the "e" from the original vitamine to create vitamin.)

Apart from where a clear-cut deficiency exists, and perhaps pregnancy, I think that there is a real possibility that doctors who prescribe vitamins as supplements, might unintentionally be giving succour to unscientific thinking.

I don't want to wax on too much, but they are no more vital than other nutrients.

If you don't get this, you're not concentrating, but I think you get my drift.

So you can understand my ambivalence when Mrs Dale asked me to recommend a good supplement.

"Ask your pharmacist for the least expensive preparation," I said, tongue-in-cheek, then rather sarcastically added, "Tell the pharmacist that it's for your dog."

She sent her domestic helper to the drugstore with a note asking for an inexpensive vitamin supplement suitable for her pet.

Imagine her surprise when he returned with

bone-shaped meat flavoured vitamin tablets!

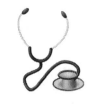

Chapter 50

The Speechless Swearing Patient

Patients may see a stony-faced doctor across the desk. Yet, he may have strong feelings, which, professionally, he cannot convey.

In the intimate space of a consultation, it's one of the toughest challenges of our profession.

I had a patient, Mrs DP, a middle-aged woman of French-Mauritian descent who was embroiled in a stormy divorce. I dreaded seeing her because of the profanities in her every sentence.

She was a woman of sharp edges, and I recoiled as she used the four-letter word in almost every sentence. I still cringe when I think about her.

I winced as she grumbled about her husband, whom she described using lurid obscenities and passed lascivious comments about their sexual relationship.

But, if you can forgive my excursion into vulgarity, I will describe a typical consultation.

(Once again, dear reader, if you are prudish, you could skip the next three paragraphs.)

"How are you today?" I asked

"I'm fine, but fucking Sandy is giving me a f... time. I wish he would go and fuck himself. You know doctor, If I could afford it, I would tell the f...ing... to f...off..."

"I have a hard time with him – and his hard on.

I winced at the double entendre.

It was unsettling, and my head spun while my vocab expanded.

I confided in my wife about the prurient Mrs DP and the cussing, expecting some guidance, but she said I was exaggerating.

So, wanting to prove my story, I decided to record our consultation. (This is illegal and unethical and I hope that if anyone from the Health Professions Council reads this, they don't strike me off the roll of medical practitioners.)

I kept a small tape recorder in the boot of my car and one Friday morning, as I entered the waiting room, I saw the lady in question waiting to see me. I returned and retrieved the recorder, which I wrapped in a magazine.

I was flustered about recording the encounter but set up the machine on the floor next to my desk, in such a way that, although the mike pointed at the patient, she couldn't see the device.

I had to press RECORD and START and then PAUSE, which would put the machine on standby. When I again pressed the PAUSE button, the machine would record to a rotating tape.

I lifted the phone, asked my receptionist to send Mrs DP in, and waited with bated breath.

As the door opened, I pressed the PAUSE button, activating the recording.

Mrs DP entered like Cruella De Ville, clacking her heels, and nattily dressed in a flamboyant Spanish-styled frock that was almost too bright to look at. She was carrying a small, satin-lined basket decorated with colourful lace. There was a little Chihuahua dog in the basket, which one only saw when it lifted its head over the rim.

As the tape rolled, there was a high-pitched weeeing sound...Weeeee...Weeee...

Ears erect (doubling its height), the dog leapt from the basket and darted to the tape recorder, sniffing vigorously!

Help! He was about to expose my clandestine operation!

I lurched forward and lifted up the dog – still sniffing the recorder.

As I lifted him, he peed on my trousers and the floor.

I reached for a nearby handful of tissues with one hand, and with the other hand thrust the dog into Mrs DP's arms!

I wiped the urine spill briskly and with a guilty expression sat back.

"How can I help you?" I squirmed.

She corrected her posture and cleared her throat. Then, with a breathy and barely audible voice, she said: "I can't talk. I've got laryngitis!"

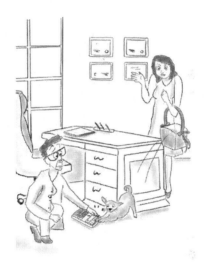

(In *101 Dalmatians*, Cruella is portrayed as the tyrannical figure in her marriage to a meek, subservient man. I wondered if Mrs DP...)

Between this chapter and the last my life took a distressing turn with a number of family tragedies which I would not want to dwell on, at the risk of spoiling the tone of this book. My intention was to entertain you with a series of humorous events, but an astute reader might be wondering why, in the earlier chapters, I did not elaborate more about my marriage and family during my GP days. I have purposely omitted these details.

So despite a childhood of poverty and great personal loss, I think the struggles I have faced have made me stronger, wiser, more compassionate and more understanding.

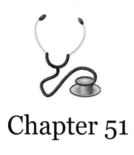

Chapter 51

The Doctor Has Left The Building – I leave General (Family) Practice

After 12 years in general practice and at 42, I felt that I should quit GP and consider a speciality. My marriage had broken up and I couldn't imagine being a family doctor without a family.

I was still interested in clinical pharmacology but couldn't see many career opportunities in that field at such a late stage in my life.

Youngsters choose from their heart, but more mature individuals use their brain. It's stunningly easy to listen to your romantic ear crying out cardiac surgery, neurosurgery or plastics – careers supposedly filled with intrigue and adrenalin, but your brain ought to tell you that these fields can leave you soul-drained. Avoiding neurosurgery was a no-brainer, and my heart was just not in cardiology. I know for a fact that most of these professionals are stressed out and disgruntled.

Many are in places where, from the outside, everybody wants to get in and, from the inside, everybody wants to get out.

I looked at the various specialities and made a spreadsheet with columns:

- Did the speciality interest me?
- What was the work-life balance?
- Did the earnings match the workload?
- How much weekend and nightwork was involved? (I had four boys to rear.)

Since much of GP involved disorders of the ear, nose and throat, ENT seemed a logical choice – especially since I had excelled in it as an undergraduate subject.

I enjoyed managing such disorders and, while no one promised it would be a day at the beach, an ENT colleague, Michael du Toit, told me that the ENT fraternity were "like one big happy family".

And that clinched it for me.

I went to see the dean at the Nelson Mandela School of Medicine in Durban.

He invited me into his office.

"Good morning Dr Desmarais," he said. "How is your

father?"

The question surprised me since my father had passed away in 1971.

"Well, he passed away some time ago," I said.

"Passed away? Oh no, that's terrible – what happened?"

I pointed out that he had taken his life in a fit of depression in December 1971.

"That's impossible!" he responded. "Your father was our family GP in Durban just a few years ago."

"That was me!" I remarked.

It was another time that my boyish looks had caused me embarrassment.

The dean advised me to take my CV to Prof. Fernandes, the head of the department of otorhinolaryngology the next day.

Prof. Fernandes was the youngest person to become a professor in South Africa. He came from Johannesburg and was very knowledgeable and highly skilled.

I knew that getting a training post at the age of 42 wouldn't be easy.

At the interview the professor said: "You are number 12 on my list. The others are above you and have certain strengths. Tell me something good about yourself and I might move you higher up the list."

I said I was conscientious and hardworking.

"That's nonsense," he said. "Everyone says that."

I told him that I got the medal for medicine in my

final year.

"Then you're a nerd," he said. "Only nerds get medals."

I told him that I had a master's degree in clinical pharmacology.

"That's the worst thing you could have told me," he said. "ENT is a surgical discipline and you'll want to use drugs to treat your patients – like a physician!"

From the sneer in his voice, I could sense the antagonism surgeons have for physicians.

"Come on," he jeered. "There must be something. You are almost off my list now!"

He flipped through my CV.

"What's this about watchmaking?" he said.

"Oh, repairing watches helped pay my way through medical school. I've got a diploma in watchmaking."

"Can you fix one of those small oblong ladies watches?"

"Uh uh, that's a 5 1/4 movement," and then, getting pally with him, I added: "Do you know that the screw that holds the hairspring is half the size of a grain of sugar?"

He smiled and then, in what I was told was probably a rare moment of self-deprecation, he joked, "So, I assume you can change the hairspring easier than I can pop in a stapes prosthesis?"

But he was obviously impressed, because my application went from the bottom of the pile to the top, and a few weeks later I started a residency (registrar training) in ENT.

I left general practice with the hilarious experiences now behind me, and probably won't write a book about life as an ENT. Specialist practice might be more demanding with pressure to make a pathologically based diagnosis.

I had a sign on my desk:

"The buck stops here."

But my watchmaking diploma sits amongst my medical qualifications as a reminder of how I secured training in otorhinolaryngology.

What were those years in general practice about?

All I know is that I was content. Not happy in that dopamine-laced, movie-ending kind of way; I just enjoyed the ride.

To love what you do and know that it matters—how could anything be more fun?

And on that note, I will leave you to ponder *why this little p...did medicine.*

Made in the USA
San Bernardino, CA
13 December 2019